PREGNANCY

FOR MODERN GIRLS

The naked truth about being pregnant

Hollie Smith

white

Important note:

The information in this book is not intended as a substitute for medical advice. Neither the author nor White Ladder can accept any responsibility for any injuries, damages or losses suffered as a result of following the information herein.

This edition first published in Great Britain 2009 by
Crimson Publishing, a division of Crimson Business Ltd
Westminster House
Kew Road
Richmond
Surrey
TW9 2ND

A catalogue record for this book is available from the British Library.

ISBN 978 1 90541 060 6

Printed and bound by the MPG Books Group

Contents

Introduction

So, you're up the duff? Well, that's wonderful news – I'm delighted for you. Having twice experienced the joy of seeing that confirmatory pink line on the pregnancy test, and spent two lots of nine months of my own life in an expectant state, I'm pretty well qualified to share in your exhilaration – not to mention your fear, nausea, pain, and extreme discomfort. And I'm really pleased to be writing this book, because it always bothered me that so many pregnancy manuals left out so much of the gory detail.

The fact is, you need the truth when you're having your first baby – and the honest truth, not the sugar-coated version. If you're likely to develop an overwhelming aversion to your husband's personal aroma, piles the size of grapes, or urinary habits that will leave you wondering if a permanent catheter is a realistic option, then better to be prepared for the possibility than to wonder WTF is going on when it actually happens and if, even in the freakish parallel universe that is being pregnant, what you're experiencing is normal. It's not just the medical stuff you need to know about, either: how, for example, is a multi-tasking modern woman supposed to carry on up the career ladder whilst pole-axed by morning sickness, or make love to her other half when she feels more like a baby elephant than a sex kitten?

Pregnancy for Modern Girls will guide you through the ups and downs of your expectant state and the birth of your baby as honestly as possible. In other words, I'm going to tell it like it is. And, rest assured, I promise to do so without any lecturing or prescribing. You're a big girl now, and you probably don't need anyone else to tell you how to behave – although you might just want some guidance so you can make up your own mind.

Whether you've been trying for a while to get pregnant or whether impending motherhood has come as something of a surprise, one thing's for sure: the next nine months are likely to be challenging, exciting and scary in equal measure. You'll just have to believe me when I say that, one day, it will all be worth it. I look at my daughters now and you know, I never, ever think about how crap I felt in the nine months I was carrying them – or even how much it hurt to squeeze the little darlings out at the end of it all. Think of it as a means to a wonderful end.

Meanwhile though, chin up. Belly out. Keep smiling. And good luck. You're going to need it.

Hollie Smith

PS There's no better source of information on a subject than someone who's already been there and done it, which is why I couldn't have written this book without help from my panel of *Modern Girls*, who regaled me with tips and tales from their own pregnancies and births and whose thoughts feature prominently throughout. My sincere thanks to them all for their commitment, their eloquence and, above all, their honesty.

Author's notes

I've referred to baby as a boy throughout and to midwives as female and doctors as male. This is pure literary licence and I apologise to all girl babies, male midwives and female doctors for my sexism ...

I've included a list of useful websites and contact numbers at the back of the book, so when I refer to an organisation, look at the back for the details.

The information in this book has been approved by midwife and mum-of-six Sara Warren.

1

You're pregnant!
What now?

His sperm's hit the target. You've got a positive test result. And the excitement (or shock, depending on your initial reaction) is starting to sink in. But what now?

WHO SHOULD YOU TELL AND WHEN?

You should probably mention it to the baby's father. And you might want to let prospective grandparents or other close relatives and good friends in on the secret. However, it's traditional to keep it largely to yourself for a while, probably because you then don't have to tell all and sundry if anything goes wrong in the more risky early months. This means that if you're ordinarily a heavy drinker or a girl who likes to let her hair down come the weekend, you'll have to think of lots of plausible reasons why you've switched to cranberry juice, or you're just not up for dancing until dawn. It was the abstinence that gave the game away in my case: walking into the pub, eight weeks gone with my first, I joined my girlfriends at the bar and requested a mineral water. Mouths dropped. A hush fell. 'Oh. My. God,' my good friend Alison responded. 'You're pregnant, aren't you?'

You don't have to tell anyone at work for quite a long time yet. Technically you can keep it to yourself until up to 15 weeks before you're due, although practically, you'll probably need to spill the beans well before that – your bump is likely to start showing once you enter the second trimester, and even before then, the fact that you keep dropping off at your desk, or disappearing to the toilet every 10 minutes will probably give the game away. There's loads more about coping with work and pregnancy in Chapter 5.

EARLY SYMPTOMS

How it feels – and how you'll look

You don't get long to adjust to the idea: within just a few weeks of conception, the hormones start to fly, as the cluster of cells inside you settles down to begin its nine-month occupancy, and your body begins the first in a whole series of very normal and natural changes. The consequences of these changes range from mildly weird to downright ghastly, some kicking in before you've even seen the little pink line on the pregnancy test. For me, it was an intense tingling in the nipples that suggested something odd was afoot. Common giveaways are sensitivity to smells, a metallic taste in the mouth, and unexplained bouts of sobbing (get used to it – you may well find yourself a gibbering wreck for the next nine months).

❝ I had really painful nipples, and was absolutely exhausted. Plus, I didn't fancy my usual glass of wine.**❞**
Jane

There's a comprehensive list of what pregnancy can do to your body in the following chapter. But early signs that you're up the duff – most of them caused by surging hormones – include:

- Tender, 'tingling', or slightly bigger boobs; darkening of the areola (the skin round the nipple).

- A heightened sense of smell or taste.

- Feeling off one or more foods or drinks, or craving something in particular. Some women say they have an odd 'metallic' taste in the mouth.

- Nausea – so-called 'morning sickness' can kick in within days of conception.

- Feeling weepy and sensitive.

- Exhaustion.

- Needing to wee a lot.

- A missed period. (Although you may still experience a little light bleeding, known as 'spotting', and this isn't necessarily anything to worry about – see page 66.)

66 I thought everything smelled 'off' – my fridge, a colleague's lunch, the inside of my car, even the carriage on the train!99
Lorna

66 Going off tea was the first sign. It made it impossible for me to hide my pregnancy from close friends and family (especially my mum) as they all wondered why I didn't want my regular cuppa.99
Laura-Jayne

GETTING USED TO BEING PREGNANT

Be prepared to take your seats on an emotional rollercoaster during the first few weeks of pregnancy (and quite possibly beyond). It's not just your body that's affected: your mind is, too. It's perfectly normal to feel a whole range of less than positive feelings, even if your pregnancy was something you planned with military precision.

You might be quite taken aback by your own fertility, especially if it happens quicker than you'd allowed for. And you're as likely to feel as terrified or indifferent as you do ecstatic. 'Excuse the term, but I was absolutely bricking it,' confesses *Modern Girl* Jenny. 'We were in no position financially to bring up a baby and I'd only just been promoted. We didn't own our own home, and we weren't married. Mostly we were terrified of telling our parents – even though we are 29 and 31!'

❝ I was actually quite horrified and spent the first month worrying that my life was over. We'd only been married four months, I was enjoying being a career girl, and I loved our third-floor flat. But then something changed and I realised it was the start of a new and very different chapter in my life. And I started looking forward to it. ❞
Lara

Men are often a little freaked out by a positive result, too (and again, this can be regardless of the fact that they impregnated you quite knowingly). My dear hubby walked around with a fixed grin that barely masked the look of terror on his face for the best part of my first pregnancy, and it's not as though he hadn't given my plans – sorry, our plans – the go-ahead.

Don't feel bad if you don't feel that good about it, at first. It's normal – most people need some time to get their head round the reality of being pregnant. Having a baby is a big responsibility, and there's no getting away from it: your life is going to change, big time. Soon, your idea of a big night out will be a 10pm dash to the garage to buy nappies and a morning that starts after 6am will constitute a lie-in. But hey, it's really not as daunting as it sounds. Reassure yourself with the knowledge that millions and millions of people have become parents before you. And lived to tell the tale.

❝ It was a surprise, as I'd only just come off the pill, and I'd assumed it would take a while. Then I felt really daunted as I thought through what it meant for our lives. It felt like our world had been turned upside down and we hadn't given it enough thought. Now I know that was madness and the timing is fine ... even if not quite the timing we would have chosen. **❞**
Sarah

GOING IT ALONE

It may have taken two of you to get pregnant, but sometimes only one of you is around to see the pregnancy through. If you're on your own (or in an unstable relationship, and likely to be that way before very long), you may be feeling even more anxious about what the future holds. Chances are you're in for a slightly harder than average pregnancy – all the difficulties, but with no-one there to support you through them. As *Modern Girl* and single mum Louise testifies, 'I knew it would probably get a bit scary on my own, but I told myself I'd stumble through on a day by day basis. It didn't stop me being really excited about my baby though – a little person who would be my whole world.'

Now's the time to draw on the support of anyone else around you who cares from among your family and friends, so that you never have to go to a scan on your own and there'll always be someone on the end of a phone at least, to commiserate if you feel sick, tired, or scared. There are also lots of organisations and websites that offer information, advice, and friendship – it's worth checking them out.

WORKING OUT D-DAY

One date is going to loom over you for the next nine months: your EDD, or estimated delivery date (sometimes just 'due date'). Your GP or midwife will work it out for you at your first appointment. You can also do the sums yourself, simply by counting 40 weeks on from the first day of your last period, which is when pregnancy is considered to start (so, somewhat oddly, you are already 'two weeks pregnant' on the day you conceive). This calculation gives you a fair idea of when you're due, but it does assume your periods follow a regular 28-day cycle which not everyone's do. Babies hardly ever arrive on their EDD anyway – less than 5% in fact.

If your periods are irregular or you haven't the foggiest when the first day of your last one was, it won't be such a simple calculation – you'll be able to find out for sure when you have your first ultrasound scan and your baby's measurements will give an accurate idea of when you're due. If this differs from the date you've already worked out, it will now be the one to go by.

THE HONEST TRUTH ABOUT DRINK AND DRUGS

66 I was mortified when I found out that I was pregnant, as the week before I 'd been out on the town three times and had drunk champagne cocktails, wine and what seemed like an entire bar 's-worth of gin, as well as smoking copious quantities of cigarettes. Whoops. 99
Lara

Lots of us find out we're pregnant quite a few weeks into pregnancy – and unknowingly have been drinking like fishes, until we realise our morning hangovers are actually morning sickness. You might feel immediately guilty for drinking before you found out, but please don't worry. Just stop the benders now!

I got very drunk before I knew. Could it have harmed the baby?

It's very unlikely. And if you didn't actually know you were pregnant when you downed all that Pinot Grigio, there's not much you can do about it, so there's definitely no point in beating your-self up.

Plenty of women have found themselves in this position – in fact, let's face it, large numbers of babies wouldn't even have been conceived if it weren't for heavy drinking sessions. Chances are you'll have caused no harm at all, although clearly it's a good idea to ease up on the drinking once you do know. However, there's nothing stopping you from sensibly enjoying the odd alcoholic beverage or two during pregnancy if it's something you enjoy (see page 88).

66 I'd been on an all-inclusive holiday, on the town with the girls and to a house-warming party before I found out, all of which had left me with a sore head. I was worried, but I knew I couldn't turn back time. I just watched everything I ate and drank from then on. 99
Marie

What about drugs?

Different drugs have different risks, but whatever it was, a one-off session is unlikely to have harmed your baby. Don't take any more though – and if you have a real problem in this area, let your midwife know and get yourself and your baby the help you need. There's more on the subject on page 94.

YOUR ANTENATAL CARE

If you haven't already, make sure you check in with a health professional at the earliest opportunity, so they can make sure you get all the antenatal care you're going to need. You can go to your GP, who'll then arrange a booking-in appointment with a midwife, or cut out the middleman and get someone at your surgery to make this appointment for you.

Systems of antenatal care vary around the country and even according to which specific clinic, surgery or hospital you attend. The care you're offered may also be influenced by choices you've made yourself, and any risk factors that may affect you.

Responsibility for keeping an eye on you may be shared between your GP and midwife, be midwife or GP-led, or, if you have any complicating factors to your pregnancy, a hospital-based consultant obstetrician will take charge overall, perhaps even seeing you in person during check-ups.

Some health authorities run what's called a domino scheme, where a whole team of community-based midwives look after you during your pregnancy, one of whom, in theory, will be with you during the birth, too. This can mean a lot of new faces over nine months.

You may be taking folic acids supplements (see page 113) already but if not, it's a good idea to start popping them as soon as you know you're pregnant.

The check-ups

You'll be offered a series of antenatal check-ups with a doctor or midwife in either a clinic, GP surgery, or at the hospital. The first of these should, ideally, take place as soon as possible, some time before the 10th week of pregnancy, since some of the tests need to be carried out before then. During this initial check-up you'll be given a whole load of information, have to answer lots of questions, and will be asked to undergo a number of tests. It's all designed to help you and your baby to good health during the pregnancy, during birth and beyond, so be as comprehensive as possible in answering and bear with all the needles and nosey questions as best you can.

It may well be the first time you've met a midwife, and you might feel a bit nervous in case she's a matronly monster, intent on telling you off for having high blood pressure and lecturing you on the evils of caffeine. It's true that plenty of women have had the bad luck to come up against a less-than-lovely midwife during their pregnancy and birth. But the vast majority are caring (if sometimes overstretched) health professionals with your best interests at heart, and even if you end up seeing one you don't like much, chances are the one you get next time will be lovely. If you *do* have a real problem with a particular midwife, however, you may be able to arrange to avoid her in the future, either by contacting your GP or your local head of midwifery services.

Subsequent appointments will be much shorter and will usually involve just urine and blood pressure checks. Regular checks on the baby will also be involved. Your abdomen will be felt to check his position and growth, and his heartbeat monitored (and even if you find antenatal check-ups a bit of a chore, it's always reassuring to hear the tiny heartbeat that reveals all is well). It's a good time to ask any questions or voice any concerns you may have. And don't forget to pipe up if you have any kind of health issue, or a family history of one, that could be relevant.

According to official guidelines, antenatal appointments should take place every four weeks until you're 28 weeks pregnant, then every three weeks until 38 weeks. You should then get one at 40 weeks and after that, if you haven't yet dropped, you'll be seen at least weekly – by which time, you'll have had enough blood pressure checks to last a lifetime and will be heartily fed up with the four walls of your midwife's office. You may not have to attend them all if there are no complications. Equally though, if anything about your pregnancy is out of the ordinary, you may be urged to present yourself more frequently.

Checking in:
what to expect at your first appointment

- You'll be asked lots of questions and may have to fill in lots of forms to help create a complete picture of your health (and your partner's), family history, work and lifestyle – all things that may in some way affect you, your pregnancy, or your baby.

- You'll be asked about where you want to have your baby.

- You'll be weighed, measured, and your BMI calculated. Your midwife needs to know if you're significantly overweight or underweight, as these could prove a complicating factor.

- You'll be asked for a urine sample (as you will on all subsequent check-ups). This can help doctors detect a number of potential problems, such as gestational diabetes (see page 109) or pre-eclampsia (see page 48).

- Your blood pressure will be taken (and at every subsequent check-up). It's common for blood pressure to rise in pregnancy and it's important to keep tabs on it because if it gets too high it's another sign of pre-eclampsia.

- A number of blood samples will be taken, to establish your blood group, check for iron-deficiency anaemia (see page 39) and for a number of infections which, whilst uncommon, could cause a problem for you or for your baby.

- You'll be given lots of other information about looking after yourself and the baby, the further tests and scans that you'll be offered, and your choices regarding your antenatal care and the birth.

You may well get to the end of your first appointment wondering if you're having a baby or applying for a job at NASA. It's a lot to take on board – still, at least you've got about another eight months or so to digest it.

WHERE ARE YOU GOING TO HAVE THE BABY?

You'll be asked early on to think about where you'd like to have the baby, and informed of what your choices are where you live. (You're entitled to go out of your area, though, if you feel strongly about it for some reason.)

Once you've decided, your doctor or midwife will 'book you in' at the unit of your choice. But you don't have to make this decision in a hurry if you don't want to – and when you do, you can still change your mind about it later in pregnancy. There are three main choices:

- A consultant-led hospital maternity unit.
- A midwife-led birthing centre if there's one in your area.
- A home birth.

There's more about the pros and cons of each on page 162.

Your antenatal notes

All pregnant women get their own personal set of antenatal notes – you'll usually be asked to keep hold of them yourself in between appointments, so you'll need to take care to bring them back for the next one, and to take them with you if you go away, just in case of a medical emergency. Do try your best not to leave them on the bus.

The notes will usually contain useful telephone numbers, and advice on what to do if anything concerns you.

If you're bewildered or concerned about the battery of tests, scans and screening that you're offered during your pregnancy, don't worry – you're not alone. To add to the confusion, not all the available antenatal tests are routinely offered in all areas, so make sure you know what you can get.

SCANS AND SCREENING

Thanks to the marvels of modern technology, you'll get at least one chance to see your baby before he's born, via ultrasound scan. For most prospective parents, this first, fuzzy glimpse of their little alien offspring is a proud and thrilling moment – even if all you can ever really make out is a jelly-like blob which bears little resemblance to anything human.

According to guidelines from the National Institute for Health and Clinical Excellence (NICE), you *should* be offered two routine ultrasound scans during your pregnancy, including one at some point between 10 and 13 weeks, usually known as the 12-week, or dating scan.

Smile, please

Most hospitals will let you take away a printout of your scan images, usually making a small charge of three or four quid. This cherished memento will give you your first chance to bore other people with your baby pictures – just don't expect them to be as excited as you are by the sight of the grainy, nondescript blob that's your son or daughter.

You may have heard about 3-D and 4-D scans, which provide an uncannily detailed image of your baby. You definitely won't get one of these scans on the NHS, so if you're keen for one, you'd need to contact a specialist service, of which there are a growing number these days.

A dating scan means your docs can firm up your EDD – or establish one, if you haven't been sure until now – by taking the baby's measurements. It will also reveal how many babies you've got in there.

Obviously in most cases, it's just the one – but around 15 in every 1,000 pregnancies results in twins, and about 150 women a year receive the gobsmacking news that they've scored a hat-trick and conceived triplets. Depending on the policy of your hospital, you may also be offered nuchal translucency screening during this scan (see below).

In spite of the fact that every pregnant women ought to get a dating scan on the NHS, there are still a few pockets of the country where they are not offered routinely and some couples who find themselves in this position choose to have one done privately for peace of mind, usually at a cost of around £100 to £150.

Whether or not you get a dating scan, you should certainly be offered one at around 18–20 weeks, by which time it's possible to see the baby in a bit more detail. This one is known as an anomaly, or mid-pregnancy scan, and is used to detect any abnormalities in the baby (although it's not guaranteed to pick up every potential problem) and to check all's well with his growth and position. The sonographer – the trained professional who carries out scans – will usually point out any visible bits of interest, like the baby's spine, and his heart, which you'll be able to see beating. You'll probably be able to make out the outline of his face, and pinpoint one or both of his hands and feet.

If anything's out of the ordinary, you may be offered more scans than are usual. And if there's something doctors want to keep an eye on, such as a low-lying placenta (see below) you should be offered at least one more scan, later on in pregnancy, to check that it's moved up.

Medical factfile: a low-lying placenta

Sometimes the placenta – the amazing organ that acts as a life support system to your baby by passing on oxygen and blood from you -- implants low in the uterus and ends up covering, or at least, threatens to cover, the cervix (the entrance to the womb). Usually, a low-lying placenta will move out of the way later on in pregnancy, in plenty of time for your baby to be born. But in about 10% of cases it won't and it then becomes known as a placenta praevia. This is a potentially risky condition, since it can cause severe bleeding, and your medical team will want to keep a close eye on you. If it's largely, or completely blocking your baby's exit route, you'll almost certainly need to have your baby by planned caesarean section (see page 184)

Does it hurt?

Nope – scans are completely painless and have no risks attached. You'll need to present yourself with a full bladder though, as it can help to push up your womb and so give a clearer picture, and given the average waiting time in a busy antenatal clinic, combined with the already dysfunctional state of most pregnant women's bladders, this can make for a pretty uncomfortable wait beforehand.

The other slight unpleasantness is the gel that's wiped across your naked tummy to help the probe glide across: it's bloody freezing.

Sonographers tend to work in silence, concentrating on seeking out all the baby's bits, and taking measurements. This can seem a little ominous, but it's normal. They'll talk you through what they can see once they're done.

Boy or girl?

Increasingly these days, it's common to find out the baby's sex at the anomaly scan. Lots of parents-to-be want to know whether they're getting the pink or the blue model – perhaps because they want to decorate and shop accordingly, decide for definite on a name, or feel it will give them a head start on the bonding process. Of course, some people are still keen for a surprise when it comes to their baby's gender and don't feel the need to know. If this is the case, though, be warned: you'll be fending off the question, 'Do you know what it is yet?' until the day when you finally do.

If you *do* want to know whether it's a girl or a boy, bear in mind that you may not be offered this information automatically, and might have to request it (pipe up at the beginning rather than the end of the scan, so there's time for the sonographer to look). There are still some hospitals where the policy is not to let on, usually because they can't guarantee it will be accurate. If they refuse and you simply *have* to know whether to go with the pink or blue on the nursery front, you might consider going private.

Remember, no-one can give a 100% guarantee of an accurate answer to this question. Once in a while, an umbilical cord gets mistaken for a willy and little Johnny turns out to be a Jane. The website of the Foetal

Anomaly Screening Programme is a good source of further information about scans.

Testing for Down's

These days, all pregnant women are offered some form of testing for Down's syndrome, a chromosomal abnormality that affects about one in every thousand babies born a year. Your risk of having a baby with Down's increases as you get older – from approximately one in 1,500 for women of 20, to one in 900 for women of 30, to one in 100 for women of 40. Testing for Down's is completely optional, and some couples don't feel the need. However, if tests establish that you *do* have a baby with Down's, you'll have time to weigh up your options – or even just to prepare for the emotional and practical needs of a child with this condition.

Initially, you'll be offered screening which won't tell you for sure whether your baby has Down's, but will indicate whether you're at high risk or not – only around 3% of tests will throw up this result, and remember, it doesn't mean for certain that your baby has Down's syndrome. Likewise, if you get a low-risk result, that doesn't mean there is no risk at all.

Screening to show the risk of Down's syndrome is done by blood test, or by ultrasound (when it's known as a nuchal translucency scan, or NT), or by a combination of both. Which type you are offered will depend on what the policy is in your area – some couples also choose to go private at this point.

If you do get a high-risk result from this initial screening, you'll be offered a diagnostic test, which will give a more definitive answer, but carries with it a slight risk of miscarriage. If it comes to this, you should get lots of support and information, as weighing up whether or not to take this option can be a tricky one. But in the end it's a personal decision, and one that only you, and your partner, can make.

There are two types of these tests available: amniocentesis, and chorionic villus sampling (CVS). Amniocentesis involves having a scan, to check the position of the baby, and a fine needle being inserted into the womb to take a sample of amniotic fluid which can then be tested. CVS is a similar process but involves taking a sample of tissue, rather than fluid, and both procedures cause some discomfort.

An amnio certainly isn't a pleasant thing to go through. 'It didn't hurt exactly, but it's very invasive – physically and emotionally,' reveals *Modern Girl* Alison. 'I glanced at the monitor only to see this enormous needle go past my son's head, which made me feel a bit giddy. It was all over before I knew it – although I could have done without the consultant waving a large test-tube full of dirty looking yellowy liquid which, he announced, was my amniotic fluid.'

On average, there's a 1% chance of miscarriage being caused by amniocentesis, and a 1%–2% chance with CVS – a risk you'll probably want to weigh up carefully before going ahead. 'There was a high risk of my son having Down's, which was why I was offered an amnio,' explains Alison. 'I blubbed for several hours, saying there was no way I would willingly have a procedure that carried a risk of miscarriage. But after the consultant explained that the risk varied from hospital to hospital, and their's was much lower than normal, I went ahead. In the end I was glad I did. The result was negative, and it meant I could relax and enjoy the rest of the pregnancy.'

You may have to wait up to a week or more for the results, and happily, in the majority of cases, they'll be negative. But if the result is a positive one, you should be offered all the advice and support you need to decide what happens next.

66 I think most women get a bit freaked out by all the scans and things they test for. It's really important to read up on everything before so you know what's going on. Once they're all done though, you can start to get really excited! 99

Lucy

Medical factfile: Down's syndrome

- Named after John Langdon Down, the doctor who first identified it, Down's syndrome is a genetic disorder that affects around one in 1,000 babies.

- A baby born with Down's is likely to have a low birth weight and a number of typical features that include slanting eyes and a flat back to the head. Physical symptoms include floppy joints and poor muscle tone. There's also an increased risk of problems with sight, hearing, heart and digestive systems.

- Children with Down's usually develop at a slower pace than is normal, and will have some degree of learning difficulties.

- There's no cure for Down's syndrome, but lots of support and treatment available that can improve health and quality of life.

When there's a problem

The majority of tests taken during pregnancy reveal all is well. But sometimes, a significant problem or potential problem is detected which can be worrying, even devastating. Should you need them, a charity called Antenatal Results and Choices (ARC) exists specifically to help people through this experience.

The test you won't get

Group B Streptococcus (Group B Strep or GBS) is a common bacterium that's carried in the vagina by around a quarter of pregnant women, usually harmlessly. However, it can be passed on from mum to baby during birth and occasionally this causes very serious problems: according to the charity Group B Strep Support, 75 babies die every year from neonatal GBS, and 40 are left with long-term health problems.

GBS can be picked up incidentally during other antenatal tests and, if this happens, you'll probably be offered antibiotics during labour, as this measure can significantly reduce the chances of your baby picking up the infection.

However, many women won't know if they're carriers or not, as screening for GBS is not carried out routinely in this country. Campaigners recommend women consider taking a test themselves through one of several private labs that offer this service. There's lots more information on the website of Group B Strep Support.

SIGNING UP FOR ANTENATAL CLASSES

A word to the wise: if you think you'd like to join the NCT and sign up for their antenatal classes, do so now. National Childbirth Trust classes are beloved by middle-class mummies-to-be the country over, and consequently they tend to fill up quicker than you can say 'natural birth' – so make contact with your local branch sooner rather than later if you're interested.

If you can't get into an NCT class, or can't afford to pay (fees range from £90 to £240 depending on where you live, although there are opportunities for subsidies), your midwife or doctor will tell you about the NHS classes available in your area, probably a bit nearer your due date. (There are also a growing number of private antenatal options, many run by independent midwives and involving luxury weekends away in classy hotels – lush, if you can afford it.)

❝ NCT classes were very useful information-wise, but it does have its share of you-must-have-a-drug-free-labour-types, so you don't get a realistic picture of how much pain labour's likely to involve. It's not helpful in the long run, as it makes women feel they've failed if they don't have the birth experience they anticipated.❞
Jane

NHS antenatal classes, often called parentcraft classes, are run by midwives and are usually pretty basic. Their availability and scheduling can also be a bit hit and miss as they tend to be subject to funding and staff cuts.

NCT classes, on the other hand, are run by specially trained teachers and take place in small group settings. It depends on the mindset of the teacher, but you'll probably notice a distinct bias with NCT-types towards natural birth and breastfeeding which, for many, is an unwelcome pressure – and you might also find there's a fair bit of showing-off going on. 'I attempted to join our nearest NCT at 12 weeks only to be told they were full. I subsequently met the group through friends anyway, only to find they were cliquey snobs – the meetings were less about the babies and more about who had the nicest house,' reveals *Modern Girl* Sheridan. Further testimony comes from Verity: 'You can fall foul of some thoroughly irritating competitive parents in the NCT, who take it all so seriously,' she agrees. 'But you can just meet up with the good ones in secret and avoid the "perfect' posse."

❝ I hated the classes. We watched a video of a birth at our first and the leader asked if we had any questions. The woman next to me put her hand up and asked if she could have a caesarean! ❞
Sara

There are pros and cons to all varieties of antenatal classes, but in most cases they're a practical way to get information and to help you prepare emotionally and practically for the birth. In particular, they can be a good way to get your man interested, if he's otherwise in denial. More importantly though, if you attend a local class you're going to meet other prospective parents there, and whilst you're bound to run into at least one other person who makes you want to stab yourself in the eyeballs, you've got a good chance of running into some like-minded folk. And you may even forge some long-term friendships.

❝ We found our NCT classes invaluable, although would have liked to have spent more time talking about caring for a baby. To be honest, the greatest value in them was the group of friends we met. ❞
Holly

Pregnancy money

If you need to find the money for antenatal classes, how about using your Health in Pregnancy Grant? This one-off payment from the government is available to all women who are 25 weeks pregnant or more. You can pick up a claim form from your midwife or doctor.

AND THE GOOD NEWS ABOUT BEING PREGNANT IS …

If all the early symptoms, reams of information, endless questions, and emotional ups and downs you're going through are getting you down, maybe it's time to remind yourself that your pregnancy is in fact a good thing. Need a few more reasons to be cheerful? How about:

- No periods for a while. Yay!

- No contraception needed, either.

- More likelihood of a seat while using public transport. (Well, once you're big enough for people to be sure they're not insulting you before offering, that is…)

- Free dental treatment. Handy if you happen to lose a crown or need a filling while you're pregnant. At the very least, make sure you get in a check-up.

- People are nice to you. (Too nice sometimes. Strangers will want to touch your belly …)

- You really need to take it easy and you certainly shouldn't be exposing your baby to all those chemicals in cleaning products … what a shame. No housework for you for a while, then.

- Great knockers. If you've already got a cracking pair this won't concern you, and will probably be an annoyance, but for the poorly endowed among us, the upgrade from A to B or more is definitely a bonus.

- You're going to need an extra 200–300 calories a day to keep your strength up. OK, so the extra calories only figure in the last trimester. But still, that's your daily Magnum justified.

- No more g-strings. Pregnancy requires big pants. Why? Because it just does, OK?

- There's shopping to be done. It might be sleepsuits and prams rather than designer shoes and new outfits, but shopping's shopping.

2

Sick and tired:
the joys of pregnancy

AILMENTS AND SYMPTOMS – HORROR STORIES OR FACTS?

OK, so what you probably want to hear about now is what pregnancy will mean for your body, other than the obvious big belly stuff. You should steel yourself for some fairly brutal truths here – pregnancy may not be an illness, but it sure does have a lot of symptoms. A massive release of hormones is to blame for most of them, coupled with the obvious physical strain of nourishing and carrying the bub. Ironically, your options for medication are limited because of potential risks to the baby, and in many cases, no-one's found an effective treatment, anyway. So pregnant women are generally expected to grin and bear whatever they're dealt. (Although I suspect that if *men* were responsible for gestation, pregnancy would entail nine months' bed rest – and someone would have invented a cure for morning sickness by now.)

As a very general rule, you can expect most of the really crap symptoms to strike during the first trimester, when the pregnancy hormones are at their most active; and the third, as the ever-expanding parasite inside you grows, kicks, grows, presses, and grows some more in the final stretch. The second trimester is the one in which all the so-called 'blooming' is supposed to take place, and certainly most women report it to be the most enjoyable bit (or rather, the least *unenjoyable* bit).

Of course, different women experience different pregnancies. You may get off lightly and suffer nothing more than a handful of minor irritations. Or you may have ticked off the whole back catalogue by the time your nine months are up. It's all down to luck, genetics … and those horrible hormones.

Here then, is a comprehensive list of the delights that can crop up during pregnancy. Be assured that these are all normal niggles (as obscure as some may seem) and, in themselves, are *usually* nothing to worry about – however much grief they're giving you. Where they *might* signal something more serious, I've said so.

Word of warning

If you're in any doubt at all about something your body's doing which it didn't do before, ask your midwife or GP. Don't feel embarrassed or silly because you want to know why your nose is bleeding, your bottom's hurting, or your veins are protruding. They're used to it. If you need an answer quickly and it can't wait, try 24-hour NHS Direct.

There are some symptoms which you should seek advice on urgently: they're listed in the box on page 65.

Morning sickness

What is it and why is it happening?

Nausea is experienced by as many as 85% of pregnant women – although 'morning sickness' is a stupid name, as it very often lasts all day. For some women it involves actual vomiting, while for others it goes no further than the distinct feeling that they're just about to. And it's horrible because it's so relentless, often going on without let-up for days, weeks and even months.

Doctors aren't really sure what causes it, although inevitably those fluctuating hormones generally get the blame. There's also an evolutionary theory: sickness is nature's way of putting pregnant women off potentially harmful foods. Either way, it can be one of the worst elements of early pregnancy, especially when it's accompanied by other symptoms such as exhaustion. Appetite is often affected; in fact, some women find they can't face food at all – and then worry about the lack of nutrition their baby is getting.

Morning sickness won't harm your baby, who'll still thrive even if you eat nothing but ginger nuts and mashed potato for three months. The good news is that it usually eases up once the first trimester is over. Morning sickness is also believed to indicate high levels of the hormone human chorionic gonadotrophin (hCG) – it's this that nourishes your baby until the placenta takes over the job at around 12 weeks and so there's a theory that morning sickness gives you a lower risk of miscarriage. (Please note, though, this is no reason to fret if you *aren't* experiencing morning sickness – not all women do.)

What can I do about it?

- Try to keep eating if you can (easier said than done) – little and often, if you can't face full meals. Experiment to try and find things that you can stomach – anything spicy or greasy is best avoided.

- If you can't eat at all, remember to drink, instead, to avoid dehydration – especially if you are actually vomiting.

- Ginger is an alternative remedy which is actually reckoned to help – try nibbling ginger biscuits, or drinking hot water infused with real ginger root.

- You could try an acupressure band, worn around the wrist, which is said to relieve nausea by pushing down on a particular pressure point. They're available from larger chemists and health food shops.

Could it be serious?

Only when it's hyperemesis gravidarum (see below). It's also important to seek help if you have vomiting that's accompanied by other symptoms, such as fever or pain, in case it's being caused by a completely different medical problem.

> **"** I had terrible morning sickness with my first and ended up taking six weeks off work. I couldn't even open the fridge door without retching and I was lucky not to end up in hospital. I survived by nibbling on plain 'white' food like bread and mashed potato. **"**
>
> Mandy

Medical factfile: hyperemesis gravidarum

Excessive vomiting in pregnancy is known as hyperemesis gravidarum. Although it's not harmful for your baby, it can cause severe dehydration that may lead to hospital treatment and, often, some weight loss. It can be really miserable particularly as it's often passed off as ordinary pregnancy nausea and therefore 'just one of those things'. However, it's important to seek out a sympathetic health professional if you're suffering, as treatment is available in the form of anti-sickness medication.

Bigger, tender boobs

What is it and why is it happening?

Changing hormones, increasing blood flow, and the beginnings of milk production all contribute to bigger boobs in the first trimester. This can be good or bad news, depending on how big they were in the first place – and unfortunately, the increase in size is often accompanied by tenderness and discomfort. Later, you may also experience a little leakage of colostrum (the creamy, first phase of milk production). You might be a bit grossed out by this, but you may as well get used to it – your boobs are going to fill up to bursting point after the birth and it's going to get a whole lot worse.

What can I do about it?

- Get yourself fitted for a new bra. Chances are you've gone up by at least a cup size so go for something as comfortable and practical as you can bear. A good bra will also help minimise sagging – an inevitable downward trend for many women.

- Get measured several times during pregnancy as your assets may swell by up to three cup sizes overall.

- If you're really big or in a lot of discomfort, you might want to wear a soft cotton sleep bra at night, too.

- A little gentle massage can ease tenderness – on the other hand, some women can't bear even to be touched.

Could it be serious?

Only for your other half, if he tries to cop a feel when they're sore.

“ I had the most incredibly sore nipples the whole way through. Nothing helped except keeping them warm, so on occasion I had no choice but to generate heat by cupping them.**”**

Jane

❝ Pregnancy destroyed my boobs. They were big and floppy, anyway, but now they're like hanging sacks. I'm seriously thinking about a boob job to sort them out.❞
Alex

Exhaustion

What is it and why is it happening?

It's common to feel absolutely knackered in the first trimester and, later on, the sheer hard work involved in carrying all that extra weight can also make you very tired. Towards the end, you could be lugging around the equivalent of up to seven bags of sugar (baby, uterus, placenta and amniotic fluid included). It can then be compounded by other common features of pregnancy such as insomnia, nausea, poor diet, or a lack of exercise. And it can be a symptom of anaemia, too, so if you're really struggling, you should chat to your midwife about it.

What can I do about it?

Not much, other than resting as much as possible, getting in as many early nights as you can, and enlisting your partner or someone else to take charge of housework and the like. You've got a damn good excuse.

Could it be serious?

No. Not unless you fall asleep in a dangerous place …

❝ I was tired, so tired that sitting down was not enough, and I'd have to lie flat for a while every day during the third trimester. Once a week throughout pregnancy I had to go to bed before 7pm: I just couldn't stay awake.❞
Helen

Indigestion and heartburn

What is it and what causes it?

Indigestion, pain or discomfort in the chest and upper tummy, and heartburn, a burning pain in the stomach, chest and throat, are extremely common during pregnancy. Hormones cause the digestive system to relax, which leads to excess acid in the stomach; and, later on, the growing womb puts pressure on the stomach.

What can I do about it?

- Try eating smaller meals, and eating slowly.

- Aim to pinpoint and cut out whichever foods are most to blame: spicy, fatty and processed foods are the usual suspects.

- Some women say drinking a glass of cold milk helps.

- If you're particularly plagued at night, try sleeping in a well propped-up position, using pillows.

- Try a suitable over-the-counter antacid remedy such as Gaviscon, which gets the thumbs up from many of the *Modern Girls*. 'I was virtually mainlining it by the end,' admits Rebecca, and both Amanda and Lara confess to 'swigging it directly from the bottle'.

Could it be serious?

No, just horribly uncomfortable. And, just to de-bunk a daft pregnancy myth, it doesn't mean you're going to have a hairy baby!

Piles

What is it and why is it happening?

Ah, piles. How thoughtful of Mother Nature to scatter this particular symptom so widely and indiscriminately among the pregnant population. Medically known as haemorrhoids, these little lumpy clusters round the back passage are caused because pregnancy hormones make the veins there swell. They can be painful, itchy, or both. They may also bleed, and will often make having a poo a wince-inducing experience (which can exacerbate the problem and cause a vicious circle if you're already suffering from constipation).

Many of the *Modern Girls* have borne this particular cross: 'Mine were as big as grapes,' says Sam. 'Mine came back with pregnancy number two and have stuck around since,' says Sheridan.

What can I do about them?

- Eat lots of fibre and drink plenty of water to keep your bowel movements loose and regular.

- An ice pack or cold flannel can provide a little relief.

- You could also ask your midwife or doctor to recommend a suitable over-the-counter cream, or, if they're severe, to prescribe suppositories.

Could it be serious?

No. But they're a right pain in the arse.

Food cravings and aversions

What is it and why is it happening?

Pregnancy cravings are the subject of many a joke. They're very real though. For *Modern Girl* Zoe it was smoked mackerel and pineapple, for Marie it was pickles and rollmops. Some women also go off certain foods, most usually caffeine, alcohol, and anything greasy or spicy. It's not really clear why either of these things happen although there are theories – they may be an evolutionary mechanism, helping to ensure a pregnant woman gets what she needs, or they may be triggered by your body's demands in the face of nutritional deficiencies.

What can I do about it?

Most cravings are harmless and can be indulged, although if you're living on a diet consisting entirely of cold baked beans or chocolate Hobnobs as a result, you should probably aim to rein it in for the good of your health.

Could it be serious?

Craving a non-food item is a psychological disorder known as pica and, unsurprisingly it isn't a good idea to consume something that's, frankly, inedible.

Among the weird items pregnant women have been known to hanker for are sand, coal, soil, soap, sponges, cigarette butts, matches, plaster, mud, sandpaper, and rubber – and you probably don't need me to tell you that none of these are good nutritional options. A yearning to chow-down on a non-edible item may be more to do with texture than taste, so you might be able to get some relief from chewing on something crunchy but innocuous, like ice.

Back pain

What is it and why does it happen?

Ever seen a heavily pregnant woman push her hands into the small of her back and wince? Back pain affects as many as three-quarters of women in pregnancy. Hormones again – this time it's something called relaxin, which is released in the body with the aim of making the joints and ligaments – especially in the pelvic region – more flexible in preparation for birth. Great, but the flipside is that it leaves your body vulnerable to pain and injury, your back included. On top of that, there's the extra weight you're carrying around the front which affects your posture for the worst.

In most cases, pregnancy back pain will ease at some point after your baby is born – unfortunately, you may find you're still suffering for a while as the effects of relaxin continue, often exacerbated by all the lifting and lugging you'll be doing once you've got a baby.

What can I do about it?

- Boring but true: regular, gentle exercise such as yoga, Pilates or swimming can help to prevent and ease backache. Strengthening your abdominal muscles is especially important, as they perform such an important role in supporting your back: try doing some pelvic tilts or 'cat' stretches daily (see page 121).

- Paying attention to your posture is vital: try to avoid standing for long periods and avoid lifting anything heavy (but if you must, make sure you bend from the knees).

- Check the position of your computer and chair, if you work at a desk.

- Ditch the high heels, as these can just make things worse.

- Try a maternity support belt, band or corset – these are made from stretchy fabric and are fixed on with straps or Velcro, with a wider panel that sits underneath the bump to give it support. You might never have considered wearing this outside of pregnancy – but may come to love it so much you're loathe to give it up once it's all over.

- Massage can help: go to a qualified professional therapist aimed at mums-to-be, or rope in your partner and get him to try some of the techniques outlined in the box below.

- If it's very bad, your doctor may prescribe pain relief medication, or refer you to a physiotherapist or other specialist.

Could it be serious?

For some women, back pain in pregnancy, especially if it's linked to pelvic girdle pain (see below), can be so severe it affects their ability to walk or move around. Let your midwife know if you're really suffering, as you can have physiotherapy.

Massage for back pain

- First find a position that's comfortable. With a bump, that's probably going to be on your side (supported with cushions if necessary), lying on a bean bag, or straddling a chair so you're facing the back of it.

- Ask your other half to apply gentle but firm circular strokes with the heels of his hand over the muscles of your lower back.

- While he's at it, get him to give your shoulders and neck a rub, too, as tension in these areas can cause or worsen pain lower down.

- Be cautious if you're using an aromatherapy oil – some aren't suitable for prengnant women, so double check first. If in doubt, stick with a little baby oil or olive oil.

Urinating (lots)

What is it and why is it happening?

Feeling the urge to wee a lot more is a symptom that can kick in early on in pregnancy: because of hormone changes, and because there's a lot more fluid in the body generally during pregnancy, as the kidneys step up a gear to rid the body of waste products.

Wee-wee overdrive usually eases up after the first trimester but often returns with a vengeance later, due to the growing pressure on the bladder caused by your expanding womb. (I remember being quite astounded that, having sat down at my desk after returning from a toilet trip, I could feel the need to go again almost immediately.)

This is often another reason for those disturbed nights. 'I've been up at least twice most nights to use the loo,' complains *Modern Girl* Liz. 'I suppose it's good practice for having a newborn.'

What can I do about it?

Not much.

- Don't be tempted to hold it in – always go with the flow, as it were.

- Make sure you've always got access to a loo.

- Aim to totally empty your bladder each time you pee, by 'rocking' backwards and forwards on the toilet a little.

- Don't be tempted to stop drinking, as we all need lots of fluids to keep us healthy – although you could try cutting them down or out late in the evening to avoid a disturbed night.

- Avoid or cut down on anything containing caffeine as it has a diuretic effect (that is, it encourages urine flow).

Could it be serious?

Not in itself, but be wary of symptoms such as bloody or cloudy wee, or pain when urinating, which could signal a urinary tract infection (UTI). It's really important to get UTIs diagnosed and treated as they're a trigger factor for premature labour (see page 189).

Abdominal pain

What is it and why is it happening?

It's not unusual to feel pains of one sort of another in your tummy during pregnancy which, although worrying, don't signal a major problem. Early on, there can a little period-like pain as the embryo implants in your womb. And a sharp, stabbing pain in the side or groin is common in the last trimester, but this is likely to be nothing more than the stretching of the muscles and ligaments around the uterus. I remember feeling horrified when I experienced these pains at one point in my first pregnancy, but a call to the midwife soon put me at ease. You may also suffer the delights of constipation, or wind (see below). And closer to D-day, 'practice' contractions known as Braxton Hicks can cause some pain or discomfort (see page 214).

What can I do about it?

It depends on the cause, but not very much. It will help if you can sit down and get some rest.

Could it be serious?

Generally speaking, tummy pains are only cause for concern if they are prolonged, or very severe, and/or you have some other symptom alongside it, such as regular, rhythmic tightening of your abdomen, bleeding, a high temperature, chills, vomiting, blood in the urine, or pain urinating. And of course, it's always possible that abdominal pain is caused by something not related to your pregnancy, such as appendicitis, which your doctor may need to rule out. Or it could simply be that you've been eating too much chocolate.

Anaemia

What is it and why is it happening?

In most cases, anaemia during pregnancy is caused by iron deficiency, which pregnant women are more prone to because of the increasing demands on their blood supply. The lack of iron means a decrease in blood cells, leading to symptoms such as exhaustion, palpitations, headaches, dizziness, and shortness of breath. It can also make you more prone to infections.

What can I do about it?

The best way to fight anaemia is by making sure you eat plenty of foods that are rich in iron (see page 111). Your GP or midwife, who'll be alert to the possibility of anaemia and may pick it up during a routine antenatal check, could suggest you take iron tablets. These often have an unwanted side effect: constipation, and you may have to try more than one sort before finding a type that suits you.

Could it be serious?

In most cases anaemia won't be a major problem, although it can make you feel pretty poorly. However, severe anaemia may increase the risk of a postpartum haemorrhage (see page 231), so your midwife or doctor might want to investigate further.

Bleeding gums

What is it and why is it happening?

Changing hormone levels cause the gums to swell and become more sensitive than usual and, in some cases, this can lead to soreness and bleeding – known as gingivitis.

What can I do about it?

- Pay careful attention to your dental care to minimise plaque, which can make the problem worse.

- Brush your teeth and gums twice daily with a fluoride toothpaste for at least two minutes (do so even if it makes them bleed more), and don't forget to floss.

- There are a couple of mouthwashes on the market which claim to help – your dentist should be able to recommend an appropriate one.

Could it be serious?

If left untreated, gingivitis can cause major decay to teeth and gums. And that won't be anything to smile about.

66 I 've had a lot of problems with my teeth this time, from gums to infected wisdom teeth that caused so much pain, but a course of antibiotics and a medicated mouthwash seemed to cure it. 99

Lucy

Smile, it's free

Don't forget that NHS dental care is free when you're pregnant, so make the most of it. You can get the exemption form you need from your midwife.

Breathlessness

What is it and what's causing it?

Many women find they're struggling to take breath at some point during pregnancy. It's very normal, and it occurs because your lungs are having to work harder to provide extra oxygen – and also when, later in pregnancy, your growing uterus pushes against your diaphragm, the muscle which helps control breathing.

What can I do about it?

Not a lot. It's normal and harmless, but if an attack of breathlessness occurs, don't panic, and try to sit down and rest for a while.

Could it be serious?

No, although it can be a sign of anaemia (see above), and you should let your midwife know if you're experiencing any other symptoms alongside, such as palpitations or chest pain.

Pain in the hands

What is it and why is it happening?

One of the slightly weirder side effects of pregnancy, the medical term for this is carpal tunnel syndrome (CPS), and it's caused by a build-up of fluid in the tube which houses the wrist nerves. It leads to variable levels of pain, throbbing, numbness or pins and needles in the hands and fingers and it commonly gets worse at night. If severe, it can affect your ability to carry out everyday tasks.

What can I do about it?

Resting and raising the hands as much as possible can help. If you're really suffering, you should be referred to a physiotherapist who may recommend wrist splints, and can give you some exercises that will help.

Could it be serious?

In most cases it eases after the baby is born. Occasionally, it persists and a minor surgical procedure is needed.

Constipation

What is it and why is it happening?

Problems with pooing commonly happen for two reasons during pregnancy: hormones relax the digestive system which slows down the movement of food through it, and your growing uterus puts pressure on your bowels and bottom. It's particularly likely to affect you if you're prone to it, anyway, or if morning sickness is preventing you from getting a balanced diet.

'The constipation in those first three months was horrendous,' recalls *Modern Girl* Alex. 'I was reduced to taking fig tablets, which would ultimately result in emergency dashes to the loo. It was most unpleasant.'

What can I do about it?

- Your best bet for tackling constipation is to get plenty of fibre-rich foods such as wholemeal bread, fruit and vegetables and pulses down you – and, crucially, drink loads of water, to help it all move through.

- Regular gentle exercise like walking and swimming will also help.

- Constipation is a common side affect of iron tablets, so if you're taking these for anaemia you could try cutting them out or switching to a different sort.

- If things get really bad, a gentle laxative treatment may help, but be sure to get advice or a prescription from your doctor or midwife as some laxatives are too strong for safe use in pregnancy.

Could it be serious?

No, although if you've also got piles it can make you seriously miserable.

Cramps

What is it and why is it happening?

Sudden spasms of pains in the legs and feet. It's not clear why they can crop up during pregnancy, but theories include muscle fatigue (other muscles in the body are working so hard to support you and the growing baby, and something has to give); a deficiency of minerals such as magnesium and potassium; and pressure on the nerves caused by the growing uterus.

What can I do about it?

- Try not to cross your legs when sitting or standing; keep your legs and ankles moving by stretching and wiggling your calves and feet whenever you get a chance.

- If you do get an attack, stretch out the leg and rotate your ankle, or try walking round the room.

- Gently rubbing the muscle can help.

- Eating a balanced diet may help boost any minerals you're missing – but check with your midwife or GP before taking any type of supplement.

Could it be serious?

No, just annoying. They'll only come in short, temporary bursts and won't last beyond pregnancy. If you've got severe, persistent leg pain and/or you're suffering from other symptoms such as swelling of the leg, contact your GP as this could be a sign of a deep vein thrombosis (see below).

Medical factfile: thrombosis

Around one or two in 1,000 women will get a blood clot in the vein during pregnancy or just after birth, when the risk is about five times higher than normal because of changes in the way the blood clots and flows. (And some people are more at risk of blood clots in general because of a genetic tendency, so you should always let your midwife or doctor know early on, if it's something that runs in your family.)

The most common sort, deep vein thrombosis (DVT), is when a blood clot occurs in a deep vein, usually in the leg. Symptoms include pain, tenderness and swelling in the leg, which may turn pale blue or reddish-purple in colour. If you notice any of these, do alert your midwife or doctor immediately.

Treatment is a medication called heparin. You could also be asked to wear compression stockings to improve blood flow and reduce swelling. It's vital to get prompt treatment for DVT, as it can lead to a dangerous complication called a pulmonary embolism, which can prove fatal.

Fainting or dizziness

What is it and why is it happening?

Your body's increased demand for blood, and later on, the pressure of the growing womb on the blood vessels can cause dizzy spells and faintness. Other factors linked to pregnancy such as tiredness, dehydration, overheating, and low blood sugar can also contribute. All in all, it's not unusual to feel wobbly and even to take a nosedive – I have a clear recollection of once doing so in the ticket queue at the tube station.

What can I do about it?

- Keep a snack on you at all times when you're out and about to give your blood sugar levels a boost if necessary.

- If you feel faint, lie down with your feet up, or sit with your head between your knees.

- Wear layers so you can avoid getting too hot, which can trigger fainting.

Could it be serious?

If it's happening a lot, you might have anaemia, and it's also a symptom of gestational diabetes. Do mention it to your midwife.

66 My blood pressure keeps dropping from time to time, leaving me a bit dizzy. In Boots recently I all but passed out while talking to the girl at the pharmacy counter. My hearing had gone completely at this point; my vision was blurred.**99**
Claire

'Baby brain'

What is it and why is it happening?

Does something happen to women's brains to make them more forgetful during pregnancy – or do they just have a lot on their mind? Science hasn't come up with an answer yet, but anecdotal evidence suggests that as many as half of pregnant women suffer from 'baby brain', or 'preg-head' as it's sometimes known.

What can I do about it?

Nothing – other than writing yourself lots of lists.

Could it be serious?

No. (Not unless one of the things you forget is to turn the gas off, or something else potentially lethal.) There's a bit more about coping with 'baby brain' at work on page 143.

66 Being a bit of a control freak, I hate the 'baby brain' effect. I can't remember what day it is, let alone whether I'm supposed to be at the midwife or the dentist. 99

Liz

Hairiness

What is it and why is it happening?

Thanks to those lovely old hormonal fluctuations, you may find that you have increased hair growth during pregnancy: usually a bonus on your head (where, it may also appear greasy, or, if you're lucky, shinier that usual) but rather less desirable over the rest of your face and body. However, some women find it works the other way and they have less body hair, or that some of the hair on their head falls out.

What can I do about it?

Up the ante on your usual depilatory regime – waxing, plucking and shaving are all fine, but do a patch test before using a hair removal cream, as skin tends to be more sensitive during pregnancy. Although there's no evidence that electrolysis and laser treatment can be harmful to a baby, some practitioners advise against it.

That said, you might find you're better off relaxing about hairier body parts – let's face it, pregnancy is one of the few times in your life when you can get away with being fat, spotty and hairy because you've got a great excuse. In any case, have you ever *tried* waxing your bikini line with a 30-week bump?

Could it be serious?

Er, no. (BTW, there's no truth in the pregnancy myth that a hairy belly means you're having a boy.)

" One benefit was that my body hair almost stopped growing. What a great side effect!"
Marie

Headaches

What causes them?
Frequent headaches are another of those common pregnancy symptoms where the cause isn't really understood. Hormones and the change in blood supply are probable culprits, and other factors like nausea and dehydration, nasal congestion, insomnia and stress may also play a part.

What can I do about it?
- If you're suffering from a headache, or can feel one coming on, try to find a moment to lie down, preferably in the dark, and rest.

- Doctors generally advise against any sort of medication in pregnancy, and aspirin and ibuprofen are out, but moderate doses of paracetamol are OK.

- If you're prone to headaches, aim for prevention rather than cure by getting as much sleep and rest as possible, eating well and drinking plenty of fluids.

- Caffeine is probably best avoided.

Could it be serious?
If you're getting many, or severe headaches or migraines, or you're having other symptoms alongside such as blurred vision, vomiting or swelling, do mention it to your midwife as there's a chance they could indicate pre-eclampsia (see below).

Medical factfile: pre-eclampsia

Raised blood pressure is very common in pregnancy, but up to one in 10 women will develop pre-eclampsia, a potentially serious form of pregnancy-related high blood pressure. It will only develop after 20 weeks and is likely to be detected during routine antenatal tests on your blood pressure and urine. Because of the risks of pre-eclampsia, you'll be closely monitored if you're found to have high blood pressure at any stage.

Symptoms of pre-eclampsia may include headaches, swelling in the hands and feet, blurred vision and vomiting. You'll be advised to eat healthily and stay active, and you may be offered medication which can reduce your blood pressure.

When pre-eclampsia becomes very severe, as it does in one or two out of every 100 women, it has serious risks as, unchecked, it can cause some potentially fatal complications, including eclampsia (convulsions); stroke; kidney failure; liver damage; and the breakdown of the body's blood clotting system. Pre-eclampsia can have serious risks for your baby too, as it can cause intra-uterine growth restriction (IGUR), and eventually, oxygen starvation.

All of which is why, if pre-eclampsia becomes severe late in pregnancy, you're likely to be admitted into hospital so you and your baby can be carefully monitored and an early delivery arranged if necessary.

Incontinence

What is it and what causes it?

Inevitably, the poor old pelvic floor muscle – which supports the bladder – comes under a lot of stress during pregnancy as the uterus grows. And it's more vulnerable than ever, because of the release of relaxin, the hormone that loosens up a pregnant woman's muscles and ligaments in preparation for birth. So, leaking wee-wee when you cough, laugh, sneeze or jump up and down, is a problem that affects many during pregnancy (and sometimes afterwards as well).

And this one's no joke: 'It was the symptom that upset me the most, I think,' admits *Modern Girl* Alex. 'I felt so ashamed that I couldn't talk to anyone about it. Sometimes I leaked without even having a cough, laugh or sneeze to blame it on and I had to wear panty-liners. I really hated it, as it made me feel old and decrepit.'

What can I do about it?

Also boring but true: the single most important thing you can do to prevent or ease the problem of a leaky bladder is regular pelvic floor exercises (see page 122). Don't be tempted to try and cut out fluids, though, as it's important to keep well hydrated for good health.

Could it be serious?

It should get better after pregnancy – but then again, birth itself can damage the pelvic floor further and for some women this results in longer term incontinence problems. All of which emphasises the importance of those wretched pelvic floor exercises. Altogether now, squeeeeze ...

66 When I was pregnant with my son, I took my daughter to the park. The walk back involved crossing a grassy area, and it was midsummer, so I had hayfever. I must have sneezed 20 times on the short walk home ... and each time I sneezed, I leaked. I had to get changed as soon as we got home. 99

Anna

Insomnia

What is it and why is it happening?

Trouble sleeping at night can be caused by any number of other pregnancy symptoms: likely culprits are back pain, overactive bladders, heartburn, and of course, that walloping great belly that's getting in the way of you and a comfy position. And since it can also be a time of high anxiety, many pregnant women find their nights are punctuated by strange dreams and wide-awake worrying.

On top of all that, unborn babies are often very active in the dead of night. So – as if to taunt you in advance of the many further nights of sleeplessness he intends to wreak upon you once born – your baby may be contributing to the problem with his insistence on paying homage to the karate kid in utero.

What can I do about it?

Make yourself as comfortable as possible with extra pillows – one between the legs and one under your bump can really help. Avoid caffeine at night. And try to get a little exercise in the evening, or at least try some relaxation and breathing techniques (see page 180).

Could it be serious?

No, just frustrating – and exhausting.

Itching

What is it and why is it happening?

Mild itching is normal and is caused because of the increased blood flow to the skin, and also, later on, as the skin stretches across your growing belly. Pregnancy hormones also make the skin more sensitive than usual, and therefore more prone generally to rashes and itchy patches.

What can I do about it?

Wear loose clothing made of natural fibres, and try using a gentle, soothing cream such as calamine lotion.

Can it be serious?

Severe itching, particularly in unusual places such as the palms of hands or soles of feet, can occasionally indicate a potentially serious liver condition called obstetric cholestasis (see below), so keep your midwife informed.

Medical factfile: obstetric cholestasis

It's not clear what causes obstetric cholestasis, a liver disorder that leads to a leakage of bile into the bloodstream.

The most common symptom, which usually doesn't develop until the third trimester, is itching; sometime mild, sometimes unbearable, and often worst on the hands and feet. But it can also cause tiredness, mild jaundice, dark urine, and a lack of appetite. Because studies in the past have linked the condition with an increased risk of stillbirth, women who are diagnosed with obstetric cholestasis are closely monitored and usually offered an induction at 37 or 38 weeks.

Obstetric cholestasis is purely pregnancy-related, and will cease to be a problem once your baby is born.

Mood swings

What is it and why is it happening?

As your nearest and dearest will no doubt vouch as they hold a bag of frozen peas to their black eye, your mood during pregnancy can be, well, changeable. Contrary to popular opinion, it's not necessarily a time of rosy glows and permanent smiles, and it's totally normal to feel intermittently miserable, since those rampaging hormones take their toll emotionally as well as physically. Naturally, you may also be worried or anxious about many things. And let's face it, if you're feeling like death thanks to the nausea, backache, or any of the other delightful symptoms outlined elsewhere in this chapter, it's just going to make things worse. 'I think the hormonal mood swings in the first trimester were probably the worst side-effect of all,' says *Modern Girl* Jenny. 'My other half would probably agree! Talk about completely irrational.'

What can I do about it?

Keep your chin up: mood swings may frequently punctuate the first trimester but will usually subside once you get into the second. Meanwhile, try to get as much rest and sleep as you can, and look for distractions in whatever makes you happy: a good book or movie, some relaxation exercises, or an evening with friends. Talk about it if you can, preferably to someone who's good at listening.

Could it be serious?

A certain amount of mood swinging is very normal, but it's known that women who feel very down during pregnancy are at higher risk of developing postnatal depression after the birth, so do mention it to your GP if you're suffering – he may refer you for counselling, or prescribe a safe form of medication.

Nose bleeds and nasal congestion

What is it and why is it happening?

The increased blood supply experienced in pregnancy, driven by your hormones, puts pressure on the veins inside the nose and causes the sinuses to swell, which makes them more prone to bleeding and/or nasal congestion (as well as snoring). As *Modern Girl* Liz reveals, 'Pretty much since I found out I was pregnant, I've had a stuffy nose and sound like I have a permanent cold.'

What can I do about it?

- If your nose bleeds, remain upright and pinch it gently but firmly for up to 10 minutes, which should stop the flow – if not, repeat.

- Take care to blow your nose gently when you need to.

- Stuffiness can be relieved with a little steam inhalation. Put a kettle full of hot water in the sink, cover your head with a towel and take a few deep breaths.

- If it gets bad, your doctor may prescribe a safe decongestant.

Could it be serious?

It's likely to be a harmless annoyance. But frequent or heavy nosebleeds can be a sign of anaemia, so if they're bad, seek help.

Overheating and hot flushes

What is it and why is it happening?

Lots of pregnant women find the switch on their natural body thermostats goes up a notch or two, caused by the increased blood flow round the body. Whilst a bit of a bonus in the winter ('I was constantly warm, which was lovely during a cold snap when our boiler broke,' reports Liz), it can add to the general misery and discomfort if you're well into pregnancy during warmer weather. And this tendency to feel the heat can sometimes come in waves, or 'hot flushes', affecting your face in particular and turning your complexion a shade of scarlet. You may find you experience some dizziness or fainting at the same time. You may also find it turns you into a bit of a sweaty Betty, as perspiring is the body's way of dealing with heat.

What can I do about it?

- Stick to loose clothing in natural fabrics, and wear layers so you can easily strip off if necessary.

- Keep the windows open for a bit of natural aircon, and consider investing in a little electric fan if you don't have air-conditioning at work.

- Don't overdo it, and don't forget to drink loads of fluids, too, as you'll find your thirst levels rise with your body temperature.

- Stay indoors, and if outside, stick to the shade.

Could it be serious?

No. Although there's evidence that a serious rise in your body temperature could be harmful to your baby, which is one reason why you're warned off saunas and very hot baths during pregnancy (see page 115 for more on that), you'd have to be very hot indeed for this to be a possibility.

66 My baby was due in early September, which was pretty bad planning in retrospect because I spent about three months of a long, hot summer desperately trying to keep cool without exposing too much of my whale-like flesh to the public at large. **99**
Maddie

Pelvic pain

What is it and why is it happening?

Thanks to the release of the hormone relaxin, the pelvic joints loosen in pregnancy to allow room for the baby's exit. Unfortunately, this increased mobility causes discomfort and/or pain in the pelvic region as well as in the buttocks, hips, legs, and lower back for many women. There may also be an audible clicking or grinding sound when you move. This condition is widely known now as pregnancy-related pelvic girdle pain or PGP. It can strike at any point in pregnancy and sometimes just afterwards.

What can I do about it?

- Good old-fashioned rest is prescribed – try to lie down whenever you can, to take the weight of body and baby off your pelvis – as is simple avoidance of the activities that hurt.

- Pay attention to your posture: aim to keep your knees close together and when standing, try to keep straight so your weight is evenly distributed over both legs.

- If PGP is causing significant discomfort or pain, your doctor may prescribe painkillers, or refer you to a physiotherapist who will suggest exercises that can help and provide equipment such as a pelvic support belt, or crutches, if necessary.

- Some women report that alternative treatments such as osteopathy provide considerable relief, so you might want to consider looking at private practitioners if you're not getting much relief from your NHS team.

Couldn't serious?

For some women, PGP can become so severe it makes ordinary activities such as walking, making love, and even turning over in bed agony. PGP can also have implications for the birth and for caring for your baby afterwards, since the symptoms can continue after pregnancy. In these cases a referral for physiotherapy will be vital. A related condition, diastasis symphysis pubis (DSP), occurs when an abnormally large gap develops between the two pubic bones at the front of the pelvis. If you need more information on pelvic girdle pain, we've included some useful addresses in the appendix at the back of the book.

❝ I started getting pelvic pain at around 14 weeks, and by 19 weeks I was having to use a mobility scooter to get into town. **❞**
Antonia

Restless leg syndrome

What it is it and why is it happening?

Restless leg syndrome (RLS) can affect anyone at any time, but doctors are unclear about its cause and why it is more common during pregnancy. It's described as an uncomfortable, sometimes painful, urge to move the legs and a feeling that your legs are 'tingling', 'crawling', or 'burning'. It usually strikes when you're resting, especially at the end of the day, so it's most likely to occur when you're sitting down in the evening or lying in bed.

Symptoms are usually eased by moving or massaging the legs but return again when you're resting – naturally, it can make it hard to get to sleep. *Modern Girl* Lara describes the problem thus: 'At seven o'clock all I want to do is sit down and watch television, but my legs have other ideas! I end up standing up in front of the telly, or pacing around the living room like a caged animal. I can't even describe the feeling really, just that my legs don't want to stay still.'

What can I do about it?
Standard advice is to try cutting out alcohol and caffeine and aim to relax in the evenings – measures you're probably taking in any case. You could try using a pregnancy pillow to support your body, while resting and sleeping. Other than that there's little you can do, unfortunately.

Could it be serious?
No – and like so many irritants of pregnancy, it will cease once you've had your baby.

Rib pain

What is it and why is it happening?
Sore and tender ribs can occur, generally later on in the third trimester, as your uterus expands and pushes against the ribs. The little Mike Tyson inside you can also cause a fair amount of pain with his kicking, punching, and head-butting. (Try not to take it personally … he's going to really love you when he gets out, honest.)

What can I do about it?
Stick to loose clothing (which you probably are, anyway), and keep an eye on your posture. A mound of well-placed cushions can aid your comfort while sitting.

Could it be serious?
No. Junior should stop using you as a punchbag once his head engages, just before birth. (See page 211).

66 With my daughter being breech, she spent the last two months head-butting my left ribs. Painful ribs were not something I thought could be so ... painful! 99
Claire

Skin changes

What is it and why is it happening?

All sorts of odd things can happen to your skin because of hormonal changes. Changes in pigmentation can cause dark patches on the face – or, if you're dark skinned, lighter patches – sometimes called 'the mask of pregnancy'.

For the same reason you may also notice moles, freckles, birthmarks, and your areolas (the skin around the nipple) darkening, and the appearance of a dark line running down the centre of your tummy – known as the 'linea nigra'.

Increased levels of blood can make your skin appear rosier than usual (hence the alleged 'blooming' or 'glowing' of women during pregnancy) and can also sometimes lead to the appearance of spider veins – small clusters of broken capillaries on the face and body. Some women find they get spotty, since hormones drive an increased production of sebum, the oily substance that keeps our skin supple.

You may also notice the appearance of skin tags, harmless blobs of excess skin which can appear anywhere on the face and body.

What can I do about it?

Not much. Most skin changes don't cause any harm, although they may look unsightly, and will fade back to normal after pregnancy. You could cover up patches, spider veins and high colour with a good foundation, and tackle oiliness with a really thorough cleansing regime.

Could it be serious?

No. It'll probably be the least of your worries.

> 66 When I was pregnant I came out in lots of red marks all over my body, especially on my face, hands and chest. They looked like burst capillaries and just appeared as little red dots. I was told that it's just a pregnancy thing. They've gone now, but were quite noticeable. 99
> Natasha

Sensitivity to smells

What is it and why is it happening?

Many pregnant women report that their sense of smell becomes very acute and that certain things (very often husbands) are suddenly emitting a pungent whiff: 'My sense of smell goes crazy during pregnancy, which means my husband gets told to leave the room when he has a beer, or Worcestershire sauce,' reveals *Modern Girl* Sara. It's thought this could be down to the same rush of hormones that (probably) cause morning sickness – and as with morning sickness, there's also a theory that it's an evolutionary thing, in place to help pregnant women automatically veer away from bad or potentially poisonous foods.

What can I do about it?

Nothing, really. If you ask your husband nicely, he will perhaps agree to station himself in another room – for the time being anyway.

Could it be serious?

No, although your other half could end up with hurt feelings.

66 One night I was woken up by a strange kind of rubbery burning smell and I thought the house was on fire. After several anxious circuits of the house, and three or four more pointless attempts to go back to sleep, I eventually tracked the smell down to a discarded carton of orange juice. Bonkers!99

Alison

Stretch marks

What is it and why is it happening?

These pink or purplish lines can appear on the belly, or anywhere else where you gain weight during pregnancy, such as breasts or thighs, and in time they fade to become silvery. They affect some women and not others: the truth is that it's all down to genetic factors that pre-determine your skin type and if you're going to get them, you're going to get them.

What can I do about them?

The only really effective solutions for stretch marks will cost you a lot of money and, for most women, it comes down to accepting them as an unavoidable symbol of motherhood – and a good splodge of fake tan. There's more about this on page 260.

Could it be serious?

Only in that your bikini days may be numbered.

66 I put tons of cream and oil on my belly, but I still ended up with a fetching wrinkly tummy from navel down, with silvery marks in the middle. I've not dared to wear a bikini yet. Not sure I ever will.99

Marie

Swollen ankles, feet and fingers

What is it and why is it happening?

Swelling in the extremities is common and is caused by displaced fluids which have been forced elsewhere in the body by the increased blood flow. It can be made worse if the weather's warm, or you've been standing for long periods.

Another reason for your feet getting bigger during pregnancy is when weight gain and softening ligaments cause your arches to drop – so your feet could easily go up a whole size or more. A bit of nuisance if it means having to purchase new (and sensible) footwear.

If you're affected, you could make like *Modern Girl* Jenny and dig out the least restrictive pair of shoes in your wardrobe: 'My feet were like balloons,' she confesses, 'but I found that flip-flops were the answer. I lived in them for the duration, rain or shine!'

What can I do about it?

- Don't stand up for too long – rest and put your feet up (literally) whenever you can.

- You can help to improve blood circulation and lessen swelling by doing some simple exercises: try rotating your foot regularly, to both sides.

- A good pair of support tights can also minimise the risks – and yes, these may sound like a garment from hell, but do try 'em before you knock 'em.

Could it be serious?

Generally, it's harmless. But keep an eye on it and mention it to your midwife (who'll be on the alert for it, in any case), as severe swelling in the hands and face can be a symptom of pre-eclampsia (see page 48).

❝ By the end of my first pregnancy I was wearing shoes three sizes too big. I didn't suffer the second time, but my feet never went back to their original size, and I was left with lots of dainty size three stilettos that I can't fit into because I'm now a four. Still, it's not like I could trip round the house wearing them with two kids under two, anyway!**❞**
Sheridan

Thrush

What is it and why is it happening?

During pregnancy, the natural balance of bacteria in the vagina is affected by hormones, which means you're up to 10 times more likely to get thrush: a yeast infection which causes a thick, creamy discharge and soreness or intense itching in and around the vagina.

What can I do about it?

- Eating natural yoghurt is said to keep thrush at bay because it contains infection-busting organisms – you can also apply it directly on your bits for some soothing (if messy) relief.

- Anti-fungal creams and pessaries are available on prescription or over the counter – some thrush treatments aren't suitable during pregnancy though, so check with your doctor or the pharmacist first.

- Meanwhile, avoid wearing tights and tight trousers, and only wear cotton pants.

- Avoid perfumed shower gels and soaps, which make the irritation worse.

- Don't forget that your partner may also need treatment in the form of cream, as thrush can be passed on sexually.

Could it be serious?

No, although it can really get you down, especially if it keeps coming back.

Vaginal discharge

What is it and why is it happening?

It's normal to have more vaginal discharge than usual during pregnancy – driven by your hormones, it's nature's way of helping to protect against infections that could travel up you to your uterus. It could also be a sign of cervical erosion (see vaginal bleeding, below). And late in pregnancy you may get a thick 'show' of discharge which could include some blood and is a sign that labour is imminent (see page 214).

What can I do about it?

Nothing, there's no need. Avoid washing with perfumed soaps or shower gels and never douche (that is, forcefully aim a jet of water up there) as it can upset the balance of chemicals in the vagina and increase your risk of infection. It it's really heavy, you can always wear a panty liner (never a tampon, for the same reason).

Could it be serious?

Keep an eye on any heavy discharge – if it becomes dark in colour or smells odd, mention it to your midwife or GP, in case you've got some kind of infection, such as thrush. A watery discharge in late pregnancy should definitely be reported: it could be leaking amniotic fluid which could signal premature rupture of the membranes (see page 189).

Varicose veins

What is it and why is it happening?

Swollen, bulgy veins that cause pain or itching are a common feature of pregnancy, as the hormones cause the blood vessels to relax and the body's increased blood flow and growing uterus put pressure on the veins. They're most common on the legs, in the anus (where they're better known as piles, see page 33), and inside the vagina. Being overweight and hereditary factors can increase your chance of suffering from them. Women carrying multiples are also more at risk.

What can I do about it?

- Put your feet up – literally. If you're suffering from swollen or aching veins in any part of your body, keeping your legs up whenever possible can help ease the pressure.

- Make sure you get regular rests if you need to stand up for work (for more on your rights at work, see Chapter 5).

- Support tights or stockings can offer some relief, while for vulval varicosities, there's something on the market called a v-brace, like a rather large pair of padded support pants.

- An ice pack (or bag of frozen peas) may prove soothing. It's also sensible to exercise gently and keep active, to boost your circulation.

Could it be serious?

No, just painful and unsightly. They'll usually go away or go down at some point after the baby's born and if not, and they're severe, it's possible to have surgery to remove them.

66 My legs have suffered, as I have varicose veins on both. No more shorts for me. 99
Amanda

Wind

What is it and why is it happening?

Bet you never thought you'd give your man a run for his money on the farting front, did you? Well, now's your chance. All those extra hormones can play havoc with a pregnant woman's digestive system – compounded later on by the pressure of the growing uterus on the stomach – and, as well as constipation and indigestion, one of the end results of this is an increase in bloating and wind. Lovely!

What can I do about it?

- Specific foods can make things worse, so you could try pinpointing the usual suspects and removing them from your diet.

- Eat small meals, and take care to chew your food before swallowing.

- Keeping active can help, too.

Could it be serious?

No. But your other half might object to the fact that you now burp more than he does.

66 Heartburn, yes. Leaky bladders, yes. And wind, yes – burps and farts after every meal. Only a minor annoyance for me. Not so nice for my husband! 99
Jane

WHEN TO GET HELP QUICKLY

Some symptoms could (although they won't necessarily) indicate a serious problem, and should be checked out as soon as possible. Get on the phone to your midwife, or make a same-day appointment with your GP, if you're experiencing one or more of the following:

- Vaginal bleeding (see the box on page 66 for more on bleeding).

- Severe, persistent abdominal pain.

- Any kind of vision disturbance.

- Sudden or severe swelling in the hands, face and eyes, especially if you also have a headache.

- A sudden raging thirst, accompanied by a lack of urination.

- Very severe vomiting coupled with pain and/or fever.

- Fluid leaking from the vagina.

- A severe headache that persists for more than a few hours.

- Pain or burning when you wee.

- Severe itching all over your body.

- A lack of foetal movements, after about 20 weeks (see page 82).

- Frequent dizziness or fainting spells.

- A heavy fall – although your baby is well cushioned inside you in his amniotic sac, it's best to be checked out after any significant knock.

If you're very concerned, and you can't get hold of a medical professional, dial 999 and ask for an ambulance.

Medical factfile: bleeding in pregnancy

The appearance of any vaginal blood can be a huge worry during pregnancy, but try not to panic if it happens to you – it's common (up to one in five pregnant women experience it) and although you should always take it seriously and get advice, in most cases it will be nothing to worry about. There may not be a cause for bleeding, but where there is, it could be:

- Implantation bleeding. Some light bleeding, usually known as 'spotting', might appear as the embryo implants in the womb, a few days after conception.

- Breakthrough bleeding. Spotting can sometimes occur at around the time your next period – and sometimes subsequent ones – would have been due.

- Cervical erosion. A condition in which the cervix is affected by cell changes which make it more prone to harmless bleeding (and not in fact because it's 'eroding' or somehow damaged, in spite of the name). It's also known sometimes as cervical ectropion. If you bleed a little after sex, it will usually be down to this. Cervical erosion may also be the cause of a heavy vaginal discharge.

- A vaginal infection. For example, vaginal thrush (see page 61), or bacterial vaginosis, which can sometimes cause a little bleeding as well as discharge, or a sexually transmitted infection such as chlamydia (see also page 157).

- An underlying cause, such as a cervical polyp (a benign growth).

- Placenta praevia. Where the placenta is low-lying in the uterus and blocks or partially blocks the cervix, from where it's more likely to detach and therefore cause bleeding, which may be severe. See also page 17.

- Placental abruption. A rare complication in which the placenta comes away from its implantation site. It will usually mean an emergency caesarean section is needed and can occasionally be life-threatening to either mum or baby.

- Spotting, or a bloody 'show' after 37 weeks could just be signs that you're close to going into labour. There's more on this on page 66.

- Sadly, bleeding does occasionally signal something very serious such as an ectopic pregnancy, where the egg has started outside the uterine cavity, most usually in the Fallopian tubes; a molar pregnancy, a very rare complication which means the fertilised egg doesn't develop into an embryo, or develops abnormally and can't survive; or a miscarriage. Although devastating, miscarriage is common, occurring in up to one in four (recognised) pregnancies, most of those in the first trimester. Usually, there's no reason – in the vast majority of cases, it's simply nature's way of dispelling a foetus that has a problem. You can get help and more information from the Miscarriage Association. Details are at the back of the book.

Do contact your midwife at the first sign of any sort of bleeding. It should always be taken seriously, and she will either be able to reassure you, or arrange for a check-up.

YOUR BABY BUMP

Whichever of the catalogue of ailments you get lumbered with, there's one that happens to all women: a dramatic change in your body's size and shape. Most women put on between 22lbs and 28lbs during a normal pregnancy. As well as a general weight gain which may see your face, bum and boobs swell to larger than normal, there'll inevitably be a rather large protuberance in the tummy area. This will gradually push out as your baby grows, and before too long you'll be the proud owner of a lovely big, firm bump. It's the most visible sign of pregnancy and, inconvenient and uncomfortable though it can be, most women feel pretty fondly about theirs as it represents the life that's growing beneath it.

Unwelcome touching

A word of warning: most women find that their big bellies prove a draw to all sorts of people (random strangers included), keen to stroke, poke, and generally comment on it. Depending on the mood you're in, this can be one of the more irritating factors about pregnancy. Try to breathe deeply and keep smiling when you come into contact with a 'prodder'. Most mean well and are merely looking to share in the miracle of life with you – they won't realise your piles are on fire and that frankly, you want to be stroked on the belly like you want your eyes poked out.

If you really can't handle it, smile, take a step back, and walk away, muttering something about your bladder calling.

Bumps can sometimes cause worry, as lots of women fret that theirs is too big, too small, or generally not doing what it's supposed to. It's important to remember that they come in all sorts of shapes and sizes, and they don't necessarily represent the size and shape your baby ends up, either.

What your bump looks like is determined by a range of factors, including:

- The size of your baby and the placenta.

- How much weight you gain.

- Your height and posture.

- The strength of your tummy muscles (the stronger they are the less noticeable your bump will be for a while, and the tighter it will be when it grows – hence in subsequent pregnancies you can generally expect to get fatter, quicker).

- How much amniotic fluid there is.

- Towards the end – the position of your baby.

- If you've got more than one baby in there, that's going to make a difference, too!

It's variable, but 12 weeks is probably the earliest you'll 'start to show', as your uterus begins to push out beyond your pubic bone from here on in. Different women will start showing at different times – if you've got a good set of abs on you, or you're very slim, you're more likely to show later than someone who isn't a gym bunny or is carrying a bit of extra weight.

66 The best bit, for a while at least, is the bump. In the second trimester I was willing it to grow, as I'd become tired of the 'Is she just fat or is she pregnant?' stage. I was desperate to get into maternity clothes – although by the end I couldn't wait to get out of them. I'd become so massive, getting my knickers on in the morning was an art. 99

Jenny

When you have your routine checks, your midwife will probably measure your bump from top to bottom with a tape measure. If so, she's looking to check the fundal height measurement, which can give a rough idea of whether or not your baby is growing at the right rate.

It's all a myth about the shape and position of your bump being a clue to the gender of your baby. Inevitably, someone will tell you that if you're carrying it 'all out the front' or 'low-slung', you've got a boy baby in there, whilst 'all round the sides' or 'carrying it high' indicates a girl. Humour them. But don't believe it.

STYLE STILL MATTERS: THE WORLD OF MATERNITY WEAR

Apart from the fact that you won't see your feet for a while, and that, for a couple of months, you'll know how it feels to be a beached whale – you'll need to re-think your wardrobe.

I'm no fashion guru, but I do understand how pregnancy and a desire to look good can sometimes seem mutually exclusive. Maternity clothing has come on in leaps and bounds in recent years and there are lots of lovely, stylish brands around. Trouble is, they can be pricey and, since you only need them for a couple of months at a time, not very cost effective. So you might have to be a bit creative – especially if you need to look good for work. Here are a few tips:

- First-off, try undoing the button and zips on your own trousers and skirts. Admittedly this will only take you to a certain point in your pregnancy, but at least it's free.

- Once this no longer works, you might want to consider investing in a 'Belly Belt' or similar – a sort of stretchy fabric waistband expander that gives you more room in your normal clothes.

- A pair of men's braces could also help keep your regular trousers up if you can't do them up any more – the 80s are back, aren't they? Hint: don't wear dungarees, though. Don't ever wear dungarees.

- Check out charity shops for good quality maternity wear, but look too at shirts, tops and skirts in a larger size than you would take normally. If you only fork out a few quid, you can donate them back again at some point after the baby's born when you're (hopefully) your old size again.

- Put out a plea on freecycle (www.freecycle.org). Someone might be looking for a new home for their old maternity wear. (It's a good place to look for other stuff, like your Moses basket, too.)

- Borrow stuff from friends who've been pregnant recently. You can always give it back if they want to extend their family later. Hint: don't be tempted to ask fat, non-pregnant friends if you can have their cast-offs…

- Check out the maternity ranges from cheap and cheerful high street chains like Peacocks and New Look.

- Invest in some good quality maternity wear basics:
  o a pair of pregnancy specific jeans, which usually come with a stretchy panel
  o a pair of black trousers
  o a smart, forgiving wrap dress
  o a couple of pretty empire line tops.

- Wear your partner's clothes. Admittedly this can go either way – a crisp, good quality work shirt worn over maternity jeans or trousers can look pretty good. A shapeless, faded T-shirt with an amusing slogan or a dodgy rock band logo across the front usually won't.

- Dress for comfort, above all else. Avoid anything with a tight waistband, plump for big cotton pants, don't dismiss maternity tights, and ditch the stilettos.

> 66 Putting my favourite skinny jeans away in the cupboard was gutting. Maternity jeans just aren't quite as stylish are they?! I bought loads of tops at the beginning of my pregnancy, but only actually wear about three. Enjoy shopping, but invest wisely. 99
> Lucy

3

Womb with a view: your baby's growth

HERE'S THE SCIENCE BIT

Bull's-eye – you've conceived! It's pretty amazing if you stop and think about it – two people, one roll in the sack, and bingo – a baby is made. In case you're interested in the science part, here's how it happens:

- Your egg, released during ovulation, and his sperm fuse together to become one cell, known as the zygote (and not to be confused with an enemy race from *Star Trek*).

- This then divides to form a cluster of cells, which travels down the Fallopian tube to your uterus (womb).

- Two or three days later, implantation occurs – in other words, the fertilised egg settles down into your womb's lining.

- At this point it becomes an embryo, and technically speaking, you're preggers – but it will be another fortnight before you're likely to suspect it, or can take a test that will let you know for sure.

And so begins a nine-month journey of astonishing growth as your baby's life begins to rapidly unfold. Each pregnancy is unique and yours may progress slightly differently from the next woman's. Babies' weight and length measurements can vary a whole lot, too. But the following gives a rough guide to what's going on inside you during those nine magical months.

Talking in weeks

Although often described as a nine-month long experience, medical folk measure the progress of pregnancy in weeks, since the changes you go through are so rapid, and it's important that specific tabs are kept on your progress. It might sound a bit faffy now, but you'll soon find yourself ticking off the time in weeks and trimesters.

HOW YOUR BABY GROWS, FORTNIGHT BY FORTNIGHT

First trimester

Pregnancy is officially dated from the first day of your last period – in other words, two weeks prior to conception. So you're already two weeks 'pregnant' before you've actually got pregnant, and by week six, the life inside you has only really been there for four weeks Confused? You will be.

At six weeks

- The tiny embryo in your uterus, safely encased in a little bag called the amniotic sac, is just 4mm–6mm in size.

- His neural tube – which will eventually become the brain and spine – has already started to develop, his vital organs are in place and his heart has begun to beat.

- He has little 'buds' where his limbs will soon be emerging, an emerging head, and dimples which will become his ears.

The placenta

Part of the cluster of cells that implanted will now develop into the placenta – the organ which links your blood supply to the baby's, and through which oxygen and nutrients are passed from you to your baby, via the umbilical cord. The same system carries waste from the baby out again. The placenta also helps protect your baby from infection as it passes on antibodies from you, and produces hormones that will sustain his growth and development in the womb.

At eight weeks

- Your baby is no longer an embryo, but a prawn-shaped foetus (the word means 'young one') and he's around 1cm–2cm long.

- Although he's bobbing around in amniotic fluid – the colourless liquid that's helping to protect him in the womb – you won't feel his movements for a while yet, although they could be detected from now by ultrasound scan.

- His face is slowly forming, too, and has small dark splodges where his eyes will be. His skin is transparent and paper-thin.

At 10 weeks

- Your baby is now around 2cm–4cm long (this is known as his crown to rump length – in other words, what he measures from head to bottom).

- He has a disproportionately large head, but his body is beginning to straighten.

- His facial features – including the beginnings of nose and upper lip – and limbs continue to grow.

At 12 weeks

- He's now fully formed. His skeleton is complete and all his body parts are in place, including the sex organs.

- He can suck, swallow, and yawn.

- He continues to be active, but you still won't feel it yet.

- His fingers and toes have separated and his hair is growing – though the colour of it could well change after he's born.

- His eyes are fully formed, but still closed, and his sense of hearing is developing.

- He already has the beginnings of his teeth – even though they won't usually make an appearance until he's five or six months old.

One trimester down ...

Getting to week 13 is a real turning point in pregnancy, because you're through the risky first trimester, when most miscarriages occur, and your chances of losing the baby become very small. It's usual to have a dating scan around now, giving you an exciting and reassuring glimpse of the bun that's in your oven.

Second trimester

At 14 weeks

- You're in the second trimester now and your baby's length is approximately 8cm–10cm.

- He has a recognisable chin, forehead and nose.

- He'll start to develop a fine covering of downy body hair, known as lanugo - which is probably there to keep him warm until he's laid down sufficient body fat to do so.

- He's already in possession of his own unique set of fingerprints.

Heartbeats

From now, your midwife may use a Doppler – a handheld ultrasound machine – to locate and listen to your baby's heartbeat. A normal foetal heart rate (FHR) can be anywhere between 110bpm and 160bpm, but on average it will be around 140–150 beats a minute - twice as fast as a normal adult's.

At 16 weeks

66 My eldest gave a mighty kick at 16 weeks and then didn't stop. She moved all day and all night. It freaked me out a bit, to be honest. 99

Jayne

- He can wave his fingers, toes and limbs around now.

- He has little fingernails in place, and he may be able to suck his thumb.

- His ears are developing and he can hear your voice, as well as your heartbeat and the rumblings and grumblings of your digestive system.

First movements

You may just about be able to make out your baby's movement from now on. At first it feels like a fluttering or bubbling sensation, very easily confused with a bout of indigestion and so often overlooked for quite a while in a first pregnancy. Don't worry if you can't feel anything yet – it's still early days, and you should pick up on them some time in the next four to six weeks.

" It took me a week or so to realise that what I thought was trapped wind was actually the first tentative kicks, at around 17 weeks. I felt so happy to feel him kick at last. "

Alison

" I felt movement in week 18, although it was initially faint 'pops' and I wasn't entirely sure what I was feeling. By week 22 they were strong enough for my husband to feel them too. They continued to come thick and fast and towards the end, when I laid down, they could be strong enough to make the duvet move. "

Mel

At 18 weeks

- He's 13cm–15cm in length now.
- He can punch kick, turn and wriggle and he may be passing the time in there by tugging and swinging on his own umbilical cord.
- His head is still large in comparison to his body, but his face is becoming more and more human in appearance. He's also pulling a range of faces.

- Although his eyes are still shut, they'll be sensitive to bright lights from outside.

- He's begun to practise his breathing skills in preparation for his exit, by inhaling and exhaling amniotic fluid.

** ❝** It's a bit weird to start with – unfamiliar, unknown, like butterfly wings. But it made me feel optimistic, happy, excited – and eager to see our baby.❞
Jane

At 20 weeks

- He's beginning to get a waxy coating known as 'vernix' to protect his skin from the soaking it's getting - most will be gone by the time he's born, but there may well be traces left.

- His hearing is well developed and he may jump or jerk at loud movements.

- His taste buds are developing.

- He'll be growing eyelashes and eyebrows.

Halfway point

You're halfway there, and you should be offered an anomaly scan now or very soon. It's usually possible for the sonographer to tell whether or not your little one is in possession of a willy (fairly accurately – but it's not guaranteed). However, you might have to ask for this information – and some hospitals still have a policy of not letting on at all.

At 22 weeks

- Your baby's crown to rump measurement will be somewhere around 18cm–20cm now.

- His head and body size will have evened out so he's in proportion – a small but perfectly formed version of the fully cooked baby you'll get to meet later on.

- He can hear and recognise your voice, so you might want to talk or sing to him – he'll find it soothing and may even give you a small kick or elbow of acknowledgement for your troubles.

At 24 weeks

- His lungs are strengthening and he'll be practising his breathing by inhaling and exhaling amniotic fluid (sometimes causing him to have hiccups, which you can feel).

- His skin will still be wrinkly, as he's yet to plump out to his full weight.

- He has fully formed eyes.

Viability

From this week, your baby is considered to be viable, which means that if born, he'd stand a chance of survival with intensive care in a neonatal unit.

At 26 weeks

- He'll open his eyes for the first time around now.

- You'll probably be well aware of all his somersaults, kicks and karate chops – unfortunately, babies in the womb often like to do most of their partying at night.

Third trimester

At 28 weeks

- His brain continues to develop and it's thought that around this time babies may begin to dream – about what, no-one knows!

- Visual responses are up and running – if you were to shine a torch at your belly, he'd turn his head to find out who put the lights on.

- His transparent skin is beginning to turn opaque.

The home stretch

Phew -- you're in your third and final trimester. Your baby's really starting to fill out your uterus and as it gets more and more crowded in there, you're likely to feel more and more uncomfortable. The reassuring news is that your baby's chances of survival, should he be born prematurely, are now very good indeed.

At 30 weeks

- Your baby should now be around 28cm long, and weighing an average 3lbs.

- His wrinkly skin will be smoothing out as he gets plumper.

- His lungs and digestive tract are almost fully formed.

66 I felt her moving bang on 16 weeks, and she was looping the loop every day afterwards. I loved the way it looked like an alien in my belly as she merrily turned over. Feeling your bubba moving is possibly the best thing about being pregnant – I missed that so much once they were out!**99**
Verity

Movement worries

You may find your baby becomes less active than he has been. It's nothing to worry about, it's just that there's less room in there for his aquarobics sessions.

Lots of mums feel huge anxiety when their babies slow down or stop moving altogether for a while, especially if they've been hyper beforehand. However, it's very normal for movement to be erratic and you probably won't need to panic. The general guideline given is that you should feel 10 or more kicks in a day, but more important than that is getting to know your baby's own pattern, so you're more likely to realise if it changes.

If you haven't felt a normal amount of movement from your baby during the period when he's usually most active, try sitting quietly for a while and drinking a glass of iced water – as your bladder fills up with chilly liquid, it should give your baby a nudge and provoke some movement. If it doesn't, and you're still concerned, let your midwife know.

66 Sometimes I would stop dead in my tracks because I couldn't remember feeling her move all day. The paranoia would get so bad, I would down glasses of iced water and prod my belly to get her to move. Then when she eventually moved the sigh of relief was huge!**99**
Jenny

66 About a week before my due date, a day went by without any movement, which was unusual. So I went into hospital, panicking. They put me on a ward and as soon as they tried to put the heart monitor round my bump the baby kicked

so hard he knocked it off! Turned out he'd just decided to have a rest that day."
Carly

At 32 weeks

- He may be lying head down in preparation for birth by now, but there's still loads of time for him to turn.

- His sleeping cycles may be longer, so you may notice he's quieter for longer periods.

- The lanugo (hair) covering his body will now begin to fall out.

Positioning is everything

Your midwife will be keeping an eye on your baby's position by feeling your abdomen carefully during your routine checks: if your baby doesn't get into pole position as you get closer to D-day, your obstetrician may carry out a procedure called an external cephalic version (ECV), to avoid a breech birth – and there are also one or two tricks you can try to encourage him round naturally (see page 210).

At 34 weeks

- Your baby now measures somewhere around 32cm in length, and weighs about 5lbs.

- He can open and close his eyelids and focus on his own fingers in front of him.

- Most of his organs are now fully mature, except for his lungs which still have a bit more developing to do.

- He's built up some fat deposits under his skin.

It's crowded in there

There's not a lot of room left in your uterus now and you may be getting prodded and poked a great deal, which can be surprisingly painful – you may find yourself cursing your little parasite.

However, it's endlessly entertaining when you can feel or see an elbow or foot protruding from your belly, alien-style, or to watch as his movements cause ripples across the surface of your tummy.

At 36 weeks

- His brain and nervous system are now fully developed and his bones beginning to harden – although the skull remains soft and flexible (hence the soft spot that your baby will have for up to 18 months after his birth) so that he can make it through the birth canal.

- If your baby is a boy, his testicles will normally have begun their descent from the abdomen into the scrotum.

- His lungs are now almost fully developed and in a week's time he'll be officially full-term. If born, he's unlikely to have any major problems and may not even need any special care.

Breech babies

Most babies will have moved into the 'head-first' position by now but a small number remain stubbornly in the 'breech' (bottom down) position, or even sideways (see page 84) – and some move round only to flip back again a bit later. You may soon feel pressure low in your abdomen, caused by the 'engagement' or 'lightening' process, as the baby drops down in preparation for birth. Some babies don't engage until the last minute, though.

At 38 weeks

- He's likely to be around 6lbs–7lbs in weight now and is definitely full-term (some experts classify 37 weeks as full-term, others 38).

- He'll have lost most or all of his hairy, waxy coatings. Gross though it sounds, he has swallowed them and will poo them out again after he's born.

- He won't be moving so vigorously – he just doesn't have the room!

On guard

It's time to be on your guard for signs of labour -- there's a more detailed guide to these on page 214.

At 40 weeks

- He's an average 35cm–37cm from crown to rump.

- He weighs anything from 6lbs–8lbs on average.

- He's got fully developed internal organs.

- He's definitely ripe and ready now. If you haven't yet gone into labour, you soon will!

Is that it?

Some pregnancies go on for 42 or even 43 weeks. Your midwife will be keeping a very close eye from now on – sometimes when a baby's procrastinating over his arrival, labour may need a helping hand (see page 215).

4

Care instructions:
eating, drinking, and other potentially 'dangerous' activities

ADAPT YOUR LIFE, DON'T DITCH IT!

Eat this, avoid that, squeeze these: it's crazy the amount of instruction you're given in pregnancy when it comes to your health and your baby's, and the list of what you should and shouldn't eat, drink, inhale, or otherwise subject your body to seems to go on forever. If you followed every one of the guidelines to the letter, you'd be carrying around a list of rules and regulations as big as your bump – and you'd be too exhausted to give birth at the end of it all.

It's true that they're all there with the best of intentions: to warn you of any potential risk (however minuscule) that something could have for your baby. Unfortunately, official guidance tends to skirt vaguely round the subject without any useful pointers as to precisely what the consequences might be, or how likely they actually are. So you end up having to choose between erring comprehensively on the side of caution (and then feeling neurotic and deprived about it), or throwing it sometimes to the wind (and then feeling rebellious and guilty).

Like lots of mums-to-be, I played it fairly safe in my first pregnancy, but took a far more fast and loose approach in my second. But neither time did I give up alcohol altogether, as is now 'officially' recommended, and I can't recall worrying about how much tea or coffee I drank. I also clearly remember tucking into a lovely bit of lightly pan-fried calves' liver (a no-no) whilst dining at a swanky London eatery one night, during my first pregnancy, on the basis that it would have been rude not to. Both my babies were perfect, thankfully – but yes, if anything had happened, I would probably have regretted every single little risk item I ever consumed, on the off-chance that it was something I could have avoided.

I can't tell you whether to be rigid or relaxed about the pregnancy rulebook. What I can do is to guide you through all the official advice, which, as you can see from the real-life opinions I've included, is advice that not everyone chooses to take. Maybe you too will decide to take the rules with a pinch of salt, or maybe you'll want to follow them to the letter, just to be sure.

The bottom line is this: we're talking guidelines here, not laws. And ultimately, the lifestyle you keep during pregnancy is down to you.

ALCOHOL

Can I have a drink during pregnancy, or not?

Until recently, pregnant women were given the official thumbs up to indulge in one or two drinks a couple of times a week. This always seemed a pretty reasonable allowance – after all, supping on the occasional glass of Merlot at the end of a long, hard day spent lugging around a big belly in the interests of procreation whilst selflessly coping with about a hundred and one unpleasant pregnancy symptoms, is hardly the action of a reckless deviant intent on causing harm to her baby.

However, in 2007, the government revised its recommendations on drinking in pregnancy, adopting the mantra that pregnant women, or women trying to conceive, should avoid alcohol altogether.

Why? Well, the truth is that doctors still aren't completely sure how much alcohol is safe to drink in pregnancy. But they know that women are drinking more heavily in general these days, that measures are bigger, and that many drinks are stronger. Hence, they've decided to hedge their bets with advice to 'play it safe' and abstain altogether.

They do know that alcohol passes from a woman's blood stream into her baby's through the placenta, and that excessive drinking could definitely be harmful. Babies born to women who drink heavily during pregnancy – in other words, anyone downing more than six units a day – are at significant risk of being born with a condition called Foetal Alcohol Syndrome, which can cause facial deformities, restricted growth, and learning and behavioural difficulties. It will also increase your risk of:

- Having a miscarriage (during the first trimester).

- Your baby's organs, nervous system and growth being affected.

- Premature birth, or a low birth weight (which means they are more vulnerable to infections and other health problems).

- Your baby being more susceptible to illness later in life.

- Suffering a stillbirth.

On the face of it, this new advice is pretty bad news for women who find it hard to face the possibility of 40 entirely dry weeks (not to mention the subsequent prolonged period of sobriety required for breastfeeding).

❝ I found it easier to not have a drink at all, rather than half a lager which then made me yearn for another,

particularly when that slightly drunken glow kicks in (usually after one lager shandy, these days)."
Alison

Fortunately, however, all the official bodies go on to point out there is no evidence that *light* drinking during pregnancy is harmful, and say that, for women who do choose to drink, a 'safe amount' is one or two units, no more than once or twice a week – in other words, exactly what the guidelines used to be.

Of course, some women find that just having one or two glasses simply leaves them yearning to finish the whole bottle and decide they'd rather cut it out altogether. But if, like me, you feel that a once or twice weekly glass of the aforementioned Merlot is better than nowt, then go ahead. And don't feel guilty about it.

" I love wine and always thought I'd struggle cutting down for nine months, but I felt so sick it was the last thing I fancied. Once the sickness went at around 20 weeks, I had five or six glasses a week, having decided that one or two units over the guidelines wasn't going to make a huge difference. I was more focused on being relaxed and happy."
Jane

What's a unit?

Wine	ABV 12%	ABV 14%
Small (125ml) glass of wine	1.5 units	1.75
Standard (175ml) glass of wine	2.1	2.45
Large (250ml) glass of wine	3	3.5

Drink	Unit
330ml bottle of 5% strength lager	1.7
Pint of 5% strength lager	2.8
25ml measure of spirit	1
35ml measure of spirit (usual amount served in pubs)	1.4
Double (50ml) measure of spirit	2
275ml bottle of alcopop (ABV 5%)	1.4

On the safe side

So the main points to remember about enjoying a tipple or two in pregnancy, are:

- You don't have to give up booze altogether. If you want to stick to the recommended 'safe levels' of alcohol during pregnancy, aim for a maximum of one to two units a week, drunk just once, or twice, per week. Some experts still reckon you should forgo booze altogether in the first trimester, though.

- When drinking, don't forget that measures these days are generous and alcohol content may be higher than you realise, so count your units and the alcohol by volume (ABV) content of your glass (see the chart below).

- Don't 'binge' drink – in other words, consume more than six units in one session (and I appreciate that may be stating the bleedin' obvious, but I mention it just in case you were thinking of getting totally ratarsed whilst knowingly pregnant...) That said, you shouldn't worry if you were drunk on the odd occasion *before* you knew you were up the duff: you're unlikely to have caused any harm as it's *prolonged* heavy drinking that's most risky.

Remember that some wines will have a higher than average ABV content, which can push the unit total up a little further. If you want to know more, there's lots of information, plus a handy online units calculator, on the website of the Drinkaware Trust.

❝ I had the odd glass of wine and the odd beer throughout, as I didn't see the harm.**❞**
Alex

CIGARETTES

Should I give up smoking when I'm pregnant?

In a word, yes. I hate to be po-faced about this, but if you smoke while pregnant, your risk of miscarriage and stillbirth increases by 26%, you're more likely to suffer some kind of complication such as placental abruption (see page 67), and there's more chance of your baby having a low birth weight (according to NHS statistics, babies of mothers who smoke are, on average, about 7oz lighter at birth than others) or being born premature, and therefore more likely to suffer infections or other health problems. Once born, your baby will be more likely to have poor lung function, and to suffer from difficulties in feeding and breathing problems like asthma, or chest and ear infections. Smoking is also one of the established risk factors for cot death – so it makes absolute sense to stop now, before you've got a baby in the house.

Does it matter that I smoked before I knew?

There's no need to worry if you smoked before you knew you were pregnant – you won't have harmed your baby in doing so because the risks outlined above are linked to pregnancies where mums have smoked throughout. As long as you stop at some point in your first trimester, your baby will be fine. The *amount* you smoke is also relevant, and even just cutting down can reduce the risks. So if you really can't stop, you should certainly aim to smoke as little as possible.

Quit while you're ahead

Pregnancy is the best excuse you'll ever have to kick the habit, and for good. Lots of women find it's a natural point at which to cut out smoking – and don't even miss it much, myself included. (I stubbed out my final 'ciggie' as soon as I found out I was pregnant the first time, and I'm glad to say I've never been tempted to take it up again since.) So if morning sickness or just general good intentions provide you with the motivation to give up, then make the most of it. And if your partner smokes, urge him to quit too: not only will it provide you with support, it will mean your home becomes smoke-free, and that's going to be so much better for your baby once born.

❝ I really wanted to smoke during my second pregnancy, but fought it off. And now I know I can resist for nine months, I'm going to keep resisting, and never go back. **❞**
Verity

There's lots of advice about giving up smoking available on the NHS website Smoke Free or by calling the NHS pregnancy smoking helpline: details for both are at the back of the book. Nicotine replacement therapy is free on prescription in pregnancy, but should only be used after appropriate advice and assessment from a health professional such as your GP or local stop smoking service specialist adviser. The sooner you can stop, the better for your baby – and for you.

❝ I used to smoke and always found it extremely hard to give up, but as soon as I found out I was pregnant I stopped straight way. I also used to like a glass of wine in the evenings and stopped that as well. The way I managed to do all of this was to stop going out altogether. **❞**
Louise

DRUGS

Regular medication

If you take regular medication for a chronic or long-term condition such as diabetes, asthma, or epilepsy, make sure your doctor knows as soon as you know that you're pregnant (that's if you haven't already sought their advice while trying to conceive). Don't stop taking your drugs without getting medical advice first, though.

Over-the-counter stuff

Pregnant women are generally advised to avoid over-the-counter medication unless it's really essential. However, you're fine to take the odd recommended dose of paracetamol, and certain essential remedies like Gaviscon, which tackles heartburn, are OK. If in doubt, ask your midwife, GP, or the pharmacist before taking or applying anything, or give NHS Direct a call (the number's listed at the back of the book). And don't assume alternative or herbal remedies will be OK because they're 'natural' – some also have risks. Again, you should check with your midwife first.

Illegal drugs

Apart from the obvious risks to your own physical and mental health, taking any sort of illegal recreational drug throughout pregnancy could certainly be harmful to your baby. While research in the area is somewhat sketchy, it's known that regular use of cannabis increases the risk of low birth weight and slow growth; speed increases the risk of congenital deformities; and taking E pushes up the risk of birth abnormalities. Cocaine is particularly dangerous stuff during pregnancy as it can trigger miscarriage, early labour, or placental abruption (see page 67) and may cause brain damage, disabilities or even death in an unborn baby.

If you did take illegal drugs on a one-off or occasional basis before you knew you were pregnant, it's unlikely to have caused your baby harm, but it's important to come clean with your doctor or midwife so they can make sure you have any additional antenatal checks that might be needed. If you have an actual drug addiction, it's vital you get it sorted out, so you'll need to tell your midwife or GP about it. They won't (or shouldn't) stand in any judgement.

CAFFEINE

Your daily brew

You'd think after all that abstinence you could at least put the kettle on and enjoy a limitless stream of your favourite hot beverage, wouldn't you? Sadly not.

The advice of the Food Standards Agency (FSA), the government's independent authority on food and nutrition, is that 200mg of caffeine is the safe daily limit to aim for in pregnancy.

That's just two mugs of instant coffee or one-and-a-half of a decent brew – and of course, caffeine can also be found in tea, cola and other soft drinks, chocolate, and certain medicines – see the list below. Reassuringly, the FSA points out that if you occasionally have more than this you shouldn't worry, as 'the risks are likely to be very small'.

> 66 If anything, my caffeine consumption was worse than ever. A work colleague used to bring me tea on the hour, every hour, to 'keep me going'. It felt too mean to just let it go cold. 99
> Lara

Fortunately for many women, nature has its own way of overturning entrenched caffeine habits (and this goes for the booze and fags, too): if you're suffering from morning sickness, the tea and coffee you previously loved may now seem about as appetising as a bowl of cold vomit.

Why is it risky?

It's thought that high levels of caffeine can increase the risk of low birth weight, making a baby more vulnerable to a range of health problems, and there's some evidence that links a very high consumption to miscarriage. Excessive amounts may also trigger or worsen a range of general health problems such as insomnia, headaches, increased blood pressure, and dehydration – all of which you could well do without when pregnant.

66 I went right off coffee with my first daughter but not so with my second, when I still had my usual two to four cups a day throughout. I now wonder if this is why the little madam is such a bad sleeper – unlike her big sister. 99
Isla

How much caffeine does it contain?

- Mug of instant coffee: 100mg
- Mug of fresh brewed or filter coffee: 140mg
- Mug of tea: 75mg
- Can of cola: 33mg
- Can of energy drink: 80mg
- 50g bar of plain chocolate: 50mg
- 50g bar of milk chocolate: 25mg
- Two-capsule dose of max strength cold and flu remedy: 50mg

66 I had issues with giving up coffee – and I like mine made like rocket fuel. I just freecycled my coffee maker, so what my eyes couldn't see... 99
Tammy

FOOD

Was it something I ate?

There are certain bugs that, if passed on to an unborn baby, could have a harmful effect on them. In pregnancy, your immune system is weakened which means you're slightly more at risk of picking up infections than usual but, even so, the chances of your baby contracting any of the infections outlined below and being harmed as a result are small. (And in some cases, it's minute).

If you *do* suspect you've contracted anything potentially harmful, you should contact your GP at the earliest opportunity, since speedy treatment can prevent the infection reaching your baby.

Raw or undercooked meat

Undercooked or raw meat can harbour the toxoplasma parasite which can cause an illness called toxoplasmosis. Most of us have already had it and are immune to it, and in a healthy adult it usually causes nothing more than mild, usually flu-like symptoms. But in a very small number of cases, (around 800 babies a year are infected, with 10% of those affected as a result) it can lead to serious illness or birth defects in an unborn child, miscarriage, or stillbirth.

- If you want to avoid the risk altogether, you should ensure your meat is well cooked, particularly poultry and minced meat products like sausages and burgers.

- Heat anything that comes from a packet until it's steaming hot all the way through.

- Pay careful attention to food hygiene where raw meat storage and preparation is concerned (see also page 107).

- It's also recommended that you avoid raw meats such as salami, pastrami and Parma ham – although these are all fine if cooked; for instance, when they're on top of a pizza.

97

Unwashed fruit, veg and salad

Soil on these things may also harbour toxoplasma, so official advice is to wash fruit, veg and salad well before eating. Some experts recommend that you do so even with the packaged, pre-washed varieties, just to be on the safe side.

Mould-ripened or blue-veined cheeses

It's advised that you forgo cheeses such as stilton, brie, camembert, Roquefort and Dolcelatte in pregnancy because they may contain listeria, a bacterium that can cause an infection called listeriosis. It's incredibly rare (infection occurs in one in 30,000 pregnancies, with the chance of harm to your baby even smaller still) and although it may result in nothing more than mild, flu-like symptoms in a pregnant woman, it can lead to serious illnesses such as meningitis, pneumonia, jaundice, premature birth, or even death in an unborn baby.

As well as avoiding the high-risk foods, you can avoid catching the listeria bug by being scrupulous about food hygiene (see the box below).

Pregnancy food myth busted!

You don't have to give up blue or squidgy cheeses completely if you don't want to. Cooking them through will remove the (already pretty small) risk of listeria, so there's nothing wrong with a bit of stilton soup or some deep-fried brie if you're hankering for a whiffy fix. You don't have to avoid all soft cheeses, either, only those that are mould-ripened or made with unpasteurised milk. So ricotta, mozzarella, mascarpone, cottage cheese and cream cheese are all absolutely fine.

---

66 I tried to avoid things I wasn't supposed to have but didn't stress too much over the odd little bit of brie, for example. As my mum said, they didn't have any

restrictions when she was pregnant with me and she ate anything she wanted. I think being happy during your pregnancy is far more important. **"**
Jane

Raw or undercooked eggs

Undercooked eggs (and poultry) may, just rarely, contain salmonella, a bacterium that causes a very nasty form of food poisoning with symptoms that include vomiting, diarrhoea, severe head and tummy pain and fever. Whilst particularly unpleasant to go through in pregnancy, it's very unlikely to cause any harm to your baby, although it can also lead to dehydration, which can cause complications. So if you've suffered a nasty bout, seek advice from your midwife or doctor.

To play safe, make sure you cook eggs through before consuming. And don't despair if you can't bear eggs boiled 'til they bounce – as long as they're lightly cooked they're fine (see below). More of a risk is anything that contains uncooked or partially cooked eggs: home-made versions of mayonnaise, Hollandaise sauce, ice cream, and certain fresh puds such as chocolate mousse, for instance – so if you're dining out, or with friends, you might want to ask first. The pre-packaged shop-brought varieties of these things are fine because they'll have been made with pasteurised eggs (in other words, heated to a point that would destroy any bacteria).

Pregnancy food myth busted!

You don't have to avoid runny or lightly cooked eggs. As long as the whites are no longer translucent, they're cooked enough to be safe. You'll also (almost certainly) be OK if you stick with the 'lion-stamped' eggs as these are inoculated against salmonella. You don't have to avoid mayonnaise, either. As long as it comes out of a jar it's fine. (And really, does anyone actually make their own?)

❝ I was a stickler about the food rules. On holiday in Corsica during my first pregnancy, I explained to a waiter that I couldn't have shellfish, steak tartare, runny cheese, and a pudding with raw eggs. He looked at me as if I was mad. On the table next to us was a hugely pregnant French lady, tucking into the entire menu and drinking red wine. But I stuck to the rules because if something had been wrong with my baby I wouldn't ever have forgiven myself. ❞

Judy

Machine ice cream

Soft ice cream that comes out of a machine is best avoided in pregnancy because it's kept at a lower temperature and there's always the risk the machine will be harbouring bacteria. Bad news if you have a penchant for Mr Whippy. Stick with ice cream from a tub, if you want to be certain.

Liver

It's thought that extremely high intake of the retinol (animal) form of vitamin A can cause birth abnormalities and since liver (and liver products such as liver pate and liver sausage) contains fairly large amounts of the stuff, the official advice is to avoid it altogether. However, as you'd need to have a pretty serious liver habit for it to be risky, you've no need to worry if you had some before you knew you were pregnant. Cod liver oil supplements also contain the retinol form of vitamin A, but not in any quantity that could be dangerous, so again, don't panic if you were taking these before you knew you were pregnant.

❝ With my first pregnancy I did exactly as I was told. But with the subsequent pregnancies I ate everything, and avoided nothing — all in moderation, of course. I figured

that in most other countries in the world, they do not have this 'dos and don'ts list' and they have perfectly normal children.**"**
Phelia

Raw (unpasteurised) milk or cheeses

These are known to sometimes harbour bacteria such as those that cause listeria, toxoplasmosis, and salmonella (see above), so you're advised to avoid them in pregnancy. Virtually all the milk and milk products you'll find in the supermarket are pasteurised, and unpasteurised milk is generally only available from specialist suppliers (it's also known as 'green top'), so it's easy enough to avoid. Goat's and sheep's milk, and their products, are often unpasteurised, so if you rely on it because of an allergy or intolerance to cow's milk, you should double check.

Pregnancy food myth busted!

Probiotic yoghurts, drinks, and other products are all perfectly safe. They do contain bacteria, but only the 'friendly' sort, which are good for us. Sour cream is fine, too.

Shellfish

It's considered sensible to avoid raw or undercooked shellfish such as prawns, mussels and oysters, as they can harbour bacteria that cause food poisoning such as salmonella (see above) and campylobacter, another very common germ. As a general rule, shellfish won't cause you any grief if you cook them before eating, or have them as part of a hot meal, but are probably best avoided from buffets where they may have been hanging around; from fish counters or stalls where you're not sure of the quality; or in ready-prepared sandwiches from sources you don't entirely trust

(you really ought to be fine if you get them from a reputable purveyor of prawn sarnies such as M&S – that's your call, though.)

Pregnancy food myth busted!

You don't have to avoid prawns altogether. They're absolutely fine if heated through (so stir fries and curries are OK) and you can also eat them cold as long as they're very fresh, they came pre-packaged and dated (rather than loose), and you eat them the same day.

❝ I was pretty bad at giving up things apart from not boozing too much. Ignored the caffeine, cheese, ham, and shellfish business totally first time round and was even more reckless second time. I think you should live your life as normal and not be too terrified of rare, rare things you might get from various foods. ❞
Rebecca

Raw fish

Advice varies on whether or not you should give up smoked salmon, trout and mackerel during pregnancy (as it's been smoked, rather than cooked, it's partially raw). The Food Standards Agency says the risk is negligible but, if you're wobbling on this one bear in mind that you'll almost certainly be fine if you stick to the stuff that comes pre-packaged and dated, and refrigerate and eat it quickly.

Sushi gets the go-head in general, as it's usually been frozen beforehand, which will kill any parasites that might be hanging around. You'll be OK if you buy it from a supermarket or make it at home (freezing it first, for 24 hours), but if you're in a restaurant, ask first to check.

Oily fish

Although generally a very nutritious food as it contains omega oils that can help prevent heart disease and may boost the development of an unborn baby's nervous system, it's advised that you don't overdo your consumption of oily fish such as fresh tuna (canned tuna doesn't count as 'oily'), mackerel, salmon, sardines, and trout, during pregnancy as they've been found to contain pollutants. Food Standards Agency guidelines recommend no more than two portions a week.

“ The nanny state has us whipped up into a frenzy of neurosis when we're pregnant. The only things I avoided completely were alcohol, caffeine and pâté. I had no problem giving up these things — in the context of my entire life it was only for a short time. But I continued to happily eat prawns, bagged salad, and stuff from Waitrose's deli counter! **”**
Nina

Fish with a high mercury content

Fish that may contain mercury, which can damage a baby's nervous system, are also best avoided: shark, swordfish, and marlin. Tuna is absolutely fine to eat in limited amounts: the FSA suggests no more than two fresh steaks or four cans of the stuff weekly.

Fresh pâté

As a fresh product which can hang around on shelves for a while but doesn't go through a heating process before consumption, pâté comes with a (tiny) risk of listeria – official advice warns against meat, fish and even vegetable varieties, although you'll be fine with those that come in a tin or are vacuum-packed. Liver pâté is a no-no anyway, because of the risks of too much vitamin A (see liver, above).

> ❝ Anything that could have caused stillbirth, like listeria in soft cheese and pâté, I gave up completely. I'm a real worrier, and would not have been able to enjoy them. ❞
> Helen

Peanuts and peanut products

Official advice on this is non-committal, as research into the matter is ongoing and authorities like the FSA and the NHS want to wait for more evidence before issuing a whole new set of guidelines. At the time of writing, both bodies say that if you're pregnant and in a high risk group (in other words, if you or your baby's dad has an allergy or an allergic condition such as eczema) you 'might want to' steer clear of peanuts and peanut products. If that's you, chat to your GP or midwife about it and do some careful research before making any decisions. We've included some sources of further information at the back of the book.

Pregnancy food myth busted!

Eating peanuts won't give your baby a peanut allergy. The jury's still out, but in fact some doctors are beginning to suspect that, if anything, early exposure to allergens may be beneficial.

You certainly don't need to avoid nuts if there is no history of allergy or allergic condition in your immediate family.

> ❝ I had a problem with not eating peanut butter in my first two pregnancies as I really fancied some. Since they're now reconsidering the evidence about peanuts and allergies, I'm enjoying my peanut butter and chicken satay this time around. ❞
> Sara

Barbecues and buffets

Bacteria breed quickly on food that's left uncovered in a warm place, so you might prefer to stick to food that's come fresh off the barbie, and be selective when it comes to party spreads, steering clear of stuff such as prawns or cold meats, for example.

Chilled, unwrapped deli foods, restaurant food, takeaways

By 'deli' foods, I mean things like cold meats, quiches, pies, salads. In strictest terms you'd give all these things up, because you just can't be certain of their hygiene history, but it would hardly be realistic. You *ought* to be fine with cold food from a reputable shop or establishment. But if you're still not convinced, the main thing to bear in mind is that anything's OK if it's been (freshly) cooked or thoroughly heated through. So that slice of deli-counter quiche is fine if you get it home and bung it in the oven for 15 minutes first, and even that takeaway meal from the slightly dodgy-looking chippie on the corner will still be OK if you actually *saw* them take the food out of the fryer and you almost burnt your mouth on it when you shovelled it in.

" I was careful in the first trimester, but got into bad habits involving runny eggs, brie, Parma ham etc., by the time I was in the second, and by the end, there was very little I wouldn't eat. Over Christmas I managed to tuck into prawn cocktail, stilton and pâté in one sitting, followed by a large Baileys. Lush. **"**
Alison

THERE'S NO POINT IN GETTING STRESSED

It's hardly surprising that so many women end up getting quite stressed over what they're supposed to avoid in pregnancy – the list goes on forever, the risks in some cases seem so minute, and advice seems to differ depending on what you're reading or who you're talking to.

Whatever you do, try not to fret too much about food safety. Play it 100% safe if it feels the right thing to do, but don't let it become a source of high anxiety. Because that's something that *definitely* isn't good for you, or your baby.

66 I was pretty neurotic about avoiding foods, medicines and anything that may harm the baby, and I've got to say it paid off as I now I have a beautiful, healthy baby. I did worry myself sick at points though, which was silly. 99
Nicola

A HEALTHY APPROACH

Why eat well?

Time for another boring-but-trueism: it makes sense to eat as healthily as possible during pregnancy. If you're eating well you'll boost your immune system and have all the energy you need to meet the extra physical demands you're under. You'll also be less likely to pile on too many excess unwanted pounds. And a good diet will also help to boost the growth and development of your baby in a number of ways. Certainly it's a good idea to steer clear of a *really* crap diet if you can: one recent study found that babies born to mums who ate lots of junk food are more likely to suffer health problems such as heart disease and diabetes later in their own lives.

Tips for good food hygiene

- Keep your kitchen clean.

- Wash your hands thoroughly before and after handling food.

- Thoroughly wash all fruit and veg.

- Defrost frozen meat and other foods thoroughly, preferably in the fridge.

- Cover food when in the fridge, and store raw and cooked products separately.

- Make sure all hot food is served piping.

- Make sure your fridge and freezer are the correct temperatures (0–4°C for fridges, below –18°C for freezers).

- Chill or freeze food as soon as you get it home from the supermarket.

- Have separate chopping boards for raw foods and foods that are ready to eat.

- Eat food within the use-by dates.

- Keep pets out of the kitchen.

OK, so eating a healthy diet in pregnancy is easier said than done. For many of us, morning sickness in the first trimester (and sometimes beyond) puts paid to a nutritious intake – or any intake at all, in some cases. I survived on a daily diet of a bread roll and a pint of milk – the only two items I could stomach – for a period of about two months in my first pregnancy. Other women have far-from nutritious food cravings that simply have to be indulged. And then, of course, there's the fact that pregnancy is a time of so few guilty pleasures. Booze, cigs and bloody red meat are off-limits. So, if you can't turn to cake, chips and chocolate in a bid to cheer yourself up, what else is there?

Beware of 'eating for two'

It's normal and natural to gain weight, and for your shape to change completely during pregnancy: you are never, ever going to have such a brilliant excuse for the pounds piling on, and you will never have a better reason for a stomach that sticks out. After all, you're growing an extra person in there, not to mention housing a ruddy great placenta and the natural resources in your breasts, to keep the said small person nourished after his birth.

However, it's worth bearing in mind that the 'eating for two' excuse is a bit of a myth – I realise this is going to make me unpopular, but I have to report that the demands of pregnancy can be met with an average increase of no more than 200–300 calories a day, and that's only in the final trimester. Shame, that. Quite apart from the extra work involved in losing your baby bulges a bit later down the line, putting on too much weight can put you at higher risk of developing conditions like pre-eclampsia (see page 48) and gestational diabetes (see below), as well as putting extra strain on your body in general and making difficulties during birth and labour more of a likelihood. And the truth is that a lot of women do put on more weight than is healthy for them in pregnancy.

So, tempting though it is to keep your spirits up by gorging on chocolate and cake, don't go overboard. There's no need to be obsessive or do anything as silly as calorie-counting – just aim for a broadly healthy diet with a good variation of different foods. In short, don't be tempted to let your food intake rocket just because you've got a baby on board, or you could be storing up future health problems for yourself. Also, you might not fit into your pre-pregnancy clothes again, ever. The galling truth is that pregnancy isn't really a licence to fill (your plate, that is).

How much weight should I gain?

It varies hugely depending on the size you started out at, but the average woman can normally expect to put on anywhere between 22lbs–28lbs. Only a third of that is accounted for by your baby – the rest is a combination of extra breast tissue, your growing uterus, the placenta, amniotic fluid, increased blood volume, extra fluid, and fat stores.

Currently, there aren't any official guidelines about what constitutes a healthy weight gain in pregnancy – experts are working on it and planning to release some soon. But in the US, they have a very general rule of thumb based on the one-two-three principle:

- If you were overweight before you got pregnant, you should aim to gain no more than one stone.

- If you were a normal weight before you got pregnant, you should aim to gain around two stone.

- If you were underweight, you should aim to gain about three stone.

Medical factfile: gestational diabetes

Being overweight or gaining lots of weight are risk factors for a pregnancy-related condition called gestational diabetes.

Diabetes occurs when the body doesn't make enough of the hormone insulin, causing high levels of blood sugar. In pregnancy you need to make more insulin for the sake of your baby, and for a small number of women, the body can't cope with this extra demand.

With gestational diabetes, you risk ending up with a very big baby and therefore a more complicated birth, with caesarean section more likely. It could also cause your baby health problems after his birth. Healthy eating and exercise is usually enough to keep blood sugar levels under control but sometimes treatment in the form of tablets or insulin injections is needed.

If in doubt, don't worry

It may be reassuring to remember that the female body is a miracle vessel that can foster new life in spite of adversity – as demonstrated by the fact that Third World mothers close to starvation can gestate, give birth to, and even feed their babies.

Do try to eat as healthily as you can, but *don't* beat yourself up if you're not consuming the perfect balance of foods you know you're supposed to.

What to aim for in a healthy pregnancy diet

- **Fruit and veg.** Five portions a day is the minimum recommended. Remember that you can include lots of things that don't really feel like fruit and veg at all: fried mushrooms, baked beans, tomato-based pasta sauces, frozen sweetcorn, strawberries and cream, and fruit smoothies, for example.

- **Starchy foods (carbs).** Aim for three or four servings of bread, rice, pasta or cereals a day, and plump for the healthier wholegrain or brown varieties whenever possible, which will help to ease constipation.

- **Protein.** Get at least two servings a day, in the form of meat, fish, eggs, beans or pulses.

- **Eat three meals a day.** As well as well-timed snacks to keep you going in between. Nutritious nibbles such as fresh and dried fruit, yoghurts and cheese, wholemeal bread or toast or a bowl of non-sugary cereal will be better for you than sweeties, cakes or crisps.

- **Calcium.** Really important for the growth and development of your baby's teeth and bones – however, you don't need any more in pregnancy than the RDA for an ordinary adult female, which is 700mg a day. That's a daily glass of milk (230mg), a pot of yoghurt (225mg) and a matchbox-sized piece of hard cheese (288mg).

Alternative sources of calcium

- Canned sardines (430mg per can)
- Bread (83mg per two slices of white or wholemeal)
- Baked beans (100mg per small can)
- Nuts such as almonds (30mg per six nuts)
- Green vegetables like broccoli (35mg per two florets)

Some products are fortified with extra calcium – certain cereals, orange juice, soya and tofu, for example – so it's always worth checking the labels.

- **Vitamin D.** This ensures your baby's bones develop well and also boosts the content in your breast milk, which is already in production. Food sources include fortified margarines, eggs, meat, and oily fish, but it's mostly provided by the sunlight we're exposed to (it's sometimes called 'the sunshine vitamin'). Some women are more vulnerable to vitamin D deficiency than others - those with dark skin, those who cover their skin, don't get out in the sunlight much, or don't get enough vitamin-D rich foods. However, the government recommends that all pregnant women take a 10 microgram (mcg) supplement of vitamin D daily.

- **Iron.** Requirements rise in pregnancy, because you're keeping your baby well supplied with it, too. Good sources of iron are red meat, leafy green vegetables like spinach, watercress and broccoli, shellfish, eggs, dried fruits like apricots or figs, nuts, pulses and beans, wholemeal bread, fortified breakfast cereals, and dark chocolate. Your doctor or midwife may suggest iron tablets if they're worried that you're seriously lacking it, but with some caution as they can cause constipation - already a prominent pregnancy side-effect for many women. There's more information about iron-deficiency anaemia on page 39.

- **Folic acid.** Taken prior to conception and during the first trimester, it can help to protect against neural tube defects such as spina bifida, a condition which can cause serious disabilities. You can get a certain amount from foods such as leafy green veg (spinach, sprouts, or greens), citrus fruits, and fortified breakfast cereals. However, official advice is to take a 400 mcg supplement of the stuff daily until your 12th week of pregnancy. Folic acid supplement tablets are readily available in chemists and supermarkets, and it's also included in most antenatal multivitamin supplements.

- **Omega 3 (or essential) fatty acids.** Reckoned to help boost your baby's brain and eyesight development. Oily fish is the best source – mackerel, sardines, kippers, salmon, fresh tuna. (Canned tuna won't cut it, as most of the healthy oils are removed in the canning process. However, tinned varieties of other oily fish such as mackerel, sardines and herrings will.) If you don't like or don't eat fish, you can get a certain amount of omega 3 from nuts and seeds.

- **Drink lots.** Water's the healthiest drink around, but you can also get your daily fluid intakes from tea and coffee (of course, there's the recommended caffeine limits to take into account), fruit juices (very high in sugars remember, so limit, drink with meals, and dilute with water where possible), and milk (which will boost your calcium intake).

Pregnancy isn't the time to be on a weight-loss diet, so any calorie-counting or carb-avoiding should definitely be ditched. If you're worried about gaining more weight than you'd wish for, simply concentrate on a broadly healthy diet as outlined above, and keep active (see the section on exercise, below).

If your diet is seriously restricted, perhaps because you're a vegan, or for a medical or religious reason, let your GP or midwife know. They may recommend a supplement, or refer you to a dietician for some extra advice.

Should I take an antenatal supplement?

The best way to get most of the nutrients we need is through the food we eat – and that means anyone who has a normal balanced diet will be fine. However, the current recommendation of the Department of Health is that all pregnant women take 400mcg of folic acid, for the first 12 weeks, and 10mcg of vitamin D, throughout pregnancy (and during breastfeeding, too). Since vitamin D isn't widely available on its own in supplement form, the only way to get a daily dose is by taking a multivitamin in which it's included. And if you're going to fork out for those, you may as well get one that also provides the folic acid, and therefore an antenatal supplement which contains both (among other stuff) is a sensible idea – especially if your diet is lacking for some reason such as prolonged morning sickness.

Antenatal supplements can be pricey, and contain lots of other things that you probably don't particularly need. Stick to supermarket or chemist own brands, which are always cheaper and are just as good. Or get hold of the Healthy Start vitamins which the government provides to pregnant women on benefits, and which contain the recommended amounts of folic acid and vitamin D, as well as some vitamin C. In some areas, you might be able to buy these very cheaply through your primary care trust (some experts think they should be routinely available to all women, anyway). It's worth asking your midwife, just in case.

If you're taking a mix of supplements rather than one single, pregnancy-specific dose, make sure you're not taking more than the recommended daily allowance of anything, as too much could be harmful for your baby.

OTHER 'DANGEROUS' ACTIVITIES

Apart from the mass of information regarding what to eat and drink, what else should be avoided in pregnancy? As with food, it's basically down to you. But here are some of the activities where a possible risk (in some cases, a very small one) has been identified:

Beauty and spa treatments

Colouring your hair

This a subject that generates lots of debate, but there's no real evidence that colouring your hair will harm your baby. Some tests have suggested it may be harmful if absorbed through the scalp and into the bloodstream, but these involved huge quantities of the chemicals in question. So, the good news for those among us who would rather spend nine months in a cupboard than let the world see our roots, is that colouring your hair in pregnancy is almost certainly safe.

It's worth bearing in mind, though, that hormonal changes affect your hair's condition so you might get a different colour or texture from the one you bargained on. You're also more likely to suffer an allergic reaction than usual, so do a strand test first.

If you're really worried and prefer to err on the side of caution, you might choose to avoid colouring your hair during the first trimester when the baby's early development takes place, as some experts recommend. Or you could stick with streaks or highlights, which aren't applied right up to the roots and so can't be absorbed into the scalp, or vegetable-based dyes. When you do dye, take the usual sensible precautions and be sure to wear gloves and apply it in a well-ventilated area. Of course, if you're suffering from morning sickness, you may find the smell of the fumes is an even worse prospect than your roots beginning to show.

Fake tan and sunbeds

Some experts say it's advisable not to use fake tan during pregnancy, but only because you're more at risk of allergic reactions – you should be fine as long as you do a patch test first. Trying to get a sunbed tan isn't a great idea, either – partly because some research links increased UV rays with folic acid deficiency, and partly because hormone levels can affect skin pigmentation, which means you may suffer from chloasma if you use a sunbed (or indeed, if you sunbathe).

Saunas, hot tubs, steam baths and Jacuzzis

Getting so hot that your body temperature rises isn't recommended, partly because it may push up the rate of your baby's heartbeat, and partly because it can affect blood pressure and cause fainting or dizziness. There's also some evidence of a link between very serious overheating and damage to your baby's nervous system.

For the same reasons, pregnant women are traditionally advised to avoid extremely hot baths, and to take care not to overdo it while exercising. So hot tubs and other such indulgences are probably best avoided, and if you're fond of a deep, hot soak, aim to keep your bath water a comfortable temperature – not so hot it turns your skin pink.

Aromatherapy

This is a great way to aid relaxation and help other pregnancy niggles, but some essential oils are believed to be unsuitable, and even potentially risky during pregnancy. Your best bet is to stick with treatment from a qualified practitioner who is registered with the Aromatherapy Council.

At home

Gardening

Because soil can contain the toxoplasmosis bug (see above), there's a tiny risk of infection if you get it on your hands. You'll be fine if you wear gardening gloves and wash your hands thoroughly when you're done.

Exposure to paints

Modern, water-based household paints (like emulsions) are safe and won't have a harmful effect on your baby. However, the NHS points out that little research has been carried out on the matter and suggests that, although if there *is* a risk it's a very small one, you avoid painting in the first trimester.

Solvent-based paints, varnishes and brush cleaners are more likely to cause harm than water-based ones, so it's recommended you don't get creative with these. It's also a good idea to avoid stripping any old paintwork since, way back before the 1970s, paint sometimes contained elements of lead, which can be poisonous.

Household chemicals and cleaning products

This is another area where there's no firm evidence of danger either way. However, it makes sense to avoid powerful products such as pesticides and oven cleaners just to be on the safe side – and let's face it, who wants to be doing cleaning when they're pregnant anyway?

Contact with animals

Cat poo has been found to harbour toxoplasmosis, so don't empty litter trays if you can help it, and use rubber gloves if you must. Bacteria is found in animal waste generally, so it's sensible to wash your hands after contact with pets.

Out and about

Mountaineering and hot air ballooning

Official advice is to avoid these two pastimes, since the high altitudes involved mean a change in oxygen levels which could potentially trigger a miscarriage. Scuba-diving is also considered a no-no during pregnancy because of some evidence that it could put an unborn baby at risk of decompression sickness (better known as the bends), and cause an increased risk of miscarriage.

Extreme sports such as hang-gliding, rock climbing, skydiving and bungee jumping

If, for any strange reason, you have a hankering for some action of this kind while pregnant, you should know that doctors warn against them –

for fairly obvious safety reasons. There's more on sports to avoid further on in this chapter, on page 124.

Theme park rides

Rapid stops and starts can damage the womb and are thus best avoided. Water slides should probably be enjoyed with caution – most pools display a warning notice to steer clear if you're expecting.

Air travel

There's no reason at all why you can't fly during an uncomplicated pregnancy, other than the fact that it may make you feel more wretched during the first trimester if you're suffering from morning sickness, and the risk that you'll go into labour later on in pregnancy. (If you've had any issues with blood pressure or bleeding, or if you have a medical condition such as diabetes, do check with your doc first.) Some airlines get twitchy about pregnant travellers from 28 weeks, and may refuse to take you, or insist on a doctor's note confirming you're fit to fly. (Policies vary, so always check before booking.) The risk of DVT (see page 44) increases when you're pregnant, so you're well advised to move around a lot during any flight, and consider wearing support stockings – low on glamour, but high on practicality.

At work

Using computers

There's no evidence of any risk to your baby as a result of regular computer use, which is a shame because it would be a darn good excuse to get signed off an office job for the duration. There's more on specific risks at work in the following chapter.

And finally … x-rays

In most cases the risk from diagnostic x-rays is low and, if you absolutely have to have one for some reason, it doesn't mean your baby will be harmed. However, doctors are likely to advise you to wait until after your baby is born if the x-ray isn't urgent. If your dentist needs to carry out a mouth x-ray, he'll provide a protective apron to wear over your belly.

Infections that could harm your baby

Some contagious infections could be harmful for your baby if you're affected by them during pregnancy, including Rubella, Chicken Pox, or Parvovirus B19 (slapped cheek disease). It's pretty unlikely you'll pick one of these up because most of us have immunity already, but if someone you've been in contact with has one and you suspect or are worried you may have caught it, do let your midwife or GP know, so they can take tests where necessary and do whatever they can to treat you and your baby.

YOU STILL NEED TO EXERCISE

Although it may be the last thing you feel like doing (particularly in the first trimester if you're feeling like crap, or in the third, when you feel huge and heavy, and you want to take a brisk stroll as much as you want to shoot yourself in the foot) it's a good idea to keep up some kind of exercise throughout pregnancy if you can.

❝ I exercised in both my pregnancies. I walked for miles, swam, and did aqua-aerobics, and I'm sure that helped me to cope after the birth. ❞
Flo

As well as boosting your general fitness, flexibility and health, exercise can aid relaxation, reduce aches and pains, improve sleep, offset constipation, and help prepare you for the physical demands of late pregnancy, labour and birth, and caring for a new baby. Research suggests that if you keep fit during pregnancy, you're more likely to have a shorter labour time and fewer delivery complications. It may also reduce the risk of developing certain pregnancy complications.

If you were a couch potato before pregnancy, now isn't the time to take up a strenuous new regime, so aim for something fairly gentle such as walking, swimming, or organised sessions specifically designed for pregnancy, such as aqua-natal classes or antenatal yoga.

If you were already fit, you can keep up the same level of activity as before for as long as you feel comfortable doing so – but bear in mind that, while it's OK to try and maintain your fitness, you definitely don't want to be training to improve it – at least, not unless you're Paula Radcliffe (and even she had to slow down a bit when expecting her daughter).

Fortunately, your body's unlikely to allow you to overdo it, so listen to what it's saying – if you're knackered, slow down or stop, and if you experience any specific problem such as bleeding or dizziness (see the full list below), get some professional advice before continuing. If you've always been a bit of a gym-obsessive, or you like to pound the pavement, you may have to accept that four or more major sessions a week are just too much right now and bring things down a notch.

You might find it hard to accept that you won't be at your physical peak for a short while, but as with all the other sacrifices of pregnancy, it's only short-term. And you don't have to give up your workout sessions entirely – just think about replacing some of them with gentler options like swimming or yoga. You may also need to reconsider certain high-impact techniques which involve lots of fast twists and turns, such as step aerobics, as your body is more vulnerable to strain and injury.

The risk of injury can be reduced by making sure you do warm up and cool down exercises either side of a workout. A decent pair of trainers, where trainers are required, is also important.

Whatever your level of fitness, you'd be wise to fit in at least a little everyday activity where possible, and to keep up your pelvic floor exercises.

Your bladder will thank you if you do (and so will your man, it's said). There's more about them below.

❝ I did a 'yoga for pregnancy' course which was amazing. I slept well afterwards and made some really good friends, too.**❞**
Jane

What sort of exercise is suitable?

Some regular aerobic (cardiovascular) exercise – in other words, the sort that raises your heart rate such as power-walking, running, dancing and low-impact aerobic classes – is fine during pregnancy if it's what your body is used to. If you never did that kind of exercise before, or if you did but now your body's asking you politely to take it down a notch, stick to walking at an ordinary (but brisk) pace, or swimming to give your heart and muscles a gentle workout.

Swimming in particular is a much-recommended way to exercise in pregnancy as the buoyancy of the water will support you and your bump and it is low impact, and therefore unlikely to leave you injured. However, the leg action of breaststroke can put pressure on the lower back and pelvis, particularly if you tend to swim with your head out of the water, so if you're suffering from pain in those areas you may be better off sticking to front or back crawl.

If getting sweaty or wet isn't your sort of thing, you may prefer to concentrate on strength conditioning exercises such as yoga or Pilates. These can improve your muscle tone and flexibility, but won't improve your cardiovascular fitness (ideally, you'd do a bit of both sorts of exercise). They're particularly good in pregnancy, as they can help to strengthen the 'core' muscles of your pelvic floor and lower abdomen, and they're particularly relaxing ways of exercising.

Look for a class designed for antenatal requirements, because there are certain positions and postures that aren't suitable when you're pregnant. (If you already go to a more general class, do at least satisfy yourself that your instructor is properly qualified, so you can get appropriate advice and adaptations for your stage of pregnancy, and make sure too that they know about your condition.) Check out the website of the Guild of Pregnancy and Postnatal Exercise Instructors to find your nearest qualified instructor.

If you fancy doing some gentle strength conditioning exercises at home, try doing some daily pelvic tilts:

- Stand with your shoulders and bottom against a wall, keeping your knees soft.

- Tilt your pelvis, so that your back flattens against the wall, and hold for about four seconds, continuing to breathe.

- Repeat up to 10 times.

Or try 'the cat':

- Get down on all fours with your hands below your shoulders and gently hold in your tummy, so that your back is flat.

- Now draw in your tummy and tilt the pelvis so that your bottom tucks under and your back rounds upwards and head curls underneath.

- Hold for a few seconds before returning to the neutral position, then repeat.

Squeezy-peasy:
the importance of pelvic floor exercises

Your pelvic floor is a layer of muscles that form a supportive 'hammock' for your bladder, bowel and uterus and, inevitably, it comes in for a massive hit whilst supporting a growing baby for nine months (and then playing a key role in its expulsion at the end of it all). It's why many women who've been through pregnancy and childbirth develop a tendency to leak urine when coughing, sneezing, exercising or laughing.

Pelvic floor exercises (sometimes called Kegels after the obstetrician who pioneered the idea) carried out regularly through pregnancy and after birth can make a real difference in preventing this. And if that's not enough incentive for you, try this: they'll help increase sensitivity during sex, and strengthen your orgasms.

The good news is that they're not difficult and you can do them any time, and any place – at your desk, watching telly, whilst washing up, etc. (The bad news is that they're rather tedious.) Here's how to do them:

- First, identify where your pelvic floor muscles are. The best way to do this is to imagine you're trying to stop weeing mid-flow (don't try this when you are actually weeing). Don't be tempted to tighten your tummy, buttock or thighs, as these aren't the muscles you're looking for.

- Try squeezing and releasing the muscles quickly, repeating up to 10 times.

- Then squeeze slowly, trying to hold the muscles tight for up to 10 seconds before relaxing. Repeat this 10 times, too.

- Ideally, you should do both sets of squeezes four to six times a day.

- A useful tip is to put little coloured stickers in various places throughout your home and in the car, as reminders to do a few squeezes when you see them. Nobody else needs to know what they're for.

> 66 I had a fantastic midwife who taught us how to do our pelvic floors by imagining you're in a lift, going up very slowly to the 20th floor. At the 20th floor you linger a bit, 'cos George Clooney's there. 99
>
> Isla

Take the stairs

Plenty of women lack time, energy or motivation to do any formal exercise when pregnant. And if you're someone who hates working out at the best of times, you're hardly likely to become a convert whilst feeling sick, heavy, or tired. Don't feel bad about it if you'd rather curl up in a ball than kick one around. Although it's true there are benefits to keeping active, many a couch-bound mum-to-be has made it through pregnancy without lifting a finger and without any untoward consequences.

If nothing else, aim to at least fit some sort of activity into your life so you don't really notice it. The best way to do this is by taking the stairs instead of the lift whenever you're presented with the choice, and by walking whenever you possibly can – the ultimate in convenient, safe, and cost-free ways to keep fit without really trying during pregnancy.

> 66 I hadn't done exercise for a long time anyway and discovering I was pregnant seemed the perfect excuse to put it off a bit longer! Lots of walking does the trick for me. That and running up escalators. 99
>
> Katie

Can exercise be risky?

The main risk in exercising during pregnancy is injuring yourself. However, there's also a very small possibility that if your body temperature shoots through the roof during the first trimester, it could damage your baby's developing nervous system. It's pretty unlikely you could work out so hard you make yourself this hot – and the body thermostat is set at a lower level than normal in pregnancy, providing a natural safety mechanism. But still, it's a good idea to drink plenty of water before, during and after exercise; to wear appropriate clothing; not to work out in very hot and humid weather, and to avoid over-exerting yourself.

Use the 'Talk Test' to give a good indication of how your body's coping: you should be able to continue a conversation whilst exercising without catching your breath.

> **“** I kept up the exercise until I started bleeding slightly and was advised to take it easy, at about six months. My pelvic floors I did at least once a day as I had a fear of my partner being disappointed afterwards.**”**
> Marie

What about my netball/riding/hockey/rugby?

If you've always keenly participated in a regular sporting activity of some kind, you may wonder if and when you should stop when you're pregnant. You'll probably know yourself how risky something feels, and how much a big, round stomach is likely to affect your balance and general prowess – so it's basically down to you whether you carry on or not. However, the experts tend to suggest you give up any type of sport that poses a significant risk of back and other injuries (weight training, rowing, tennis), losing your balance and falling (gymnastics, ice hockey, skiing, cycling, horse-riding), or being inadvertently walloped (kickboxing, judo, football, rugby). You may find that once you've got a baby inside you, your keenness for these kinds of things will waver, in any case.

When you shouldn't exercise

Exercise may not be a good idea if you have a chronic condition or if your pregnancy is affected by any sort of complication – if one develops, you might have to stop. If in any doubt, check with your doctor or midwife. Generally speaking, you should stop exercising and seek prompt advice if you experience one or more of the following symptoms:

- Dizziness or feeling faint.
- Headache.
- Shortness of breath on exertion.
- Difficulty in getting your breath while exercising.
- Pain or palpitations in your chest.
- Pain in your abdomen, back or pubic area, or in your pelvic girdle.
- Weakness in your muscles.
- Pain or swelling in your leg(s).
- Painful uterine contractions.
- Fewer movements from your baby.
- Leakage of your amniotic fluids.
- Bleeding.

5

Office politics:
pregnancy and your career

YOUR RIGHTS AND RESPONSIBILITIES

This chapter covers a dull subject – full of legislation and government rules. It's very easy to get bogged down in this (or so bored you don't pay attention). That said, it is very important to be aware of your rights, and what's offered to you, so I've tried to lay it out in plain English.

However important your career is to you, being pregnant can really take the shine off your working day. In some women's ideal world, you'd be given the whole nine months off, paid. Others are happy to work right up to labour and find the pregnancy a rather annoying blip in your career climb.

Of course, it's not an ideal world – but there are choices to be made. In most cases maternity leave won't begin until a month or so before your due date, if not later, and until then you must simply plough on at work, whilst doing your best to tackle the full range of physical and mental disadvantages that pregnancy wreaks.

You might also feel a bit wobbly about your impending maternity leave, wondering who's going to keep things running smoothly in your role while you're gone, or worse, that the person who does take over turns out to be better at it than you are. Maybe you're having to kiss goodbye to that promotion you've been working towards – or even fear this could be the end of your career entirely. These are all very understandable concerns – although personally I couldn't wait to leave my job and had no intention of going back: I've seen a number of friends put flourishing careers aside for their babies, only to struggle to pick up the pieces afterwards.

The attitude of your boss and your colleagues will inevitably affect how you cope with your career during pregnancy. If we did all live in that ideal world, every pregnant woman would have the respect, support, and sympathy of her manager and fellow workers – and sadly, for some, the reality is rather different.

When to tell your boss the news

You don't have to tell your boss that you're pregnant for quite a while, if you don't want to – but you must have done so before you're 25 weeks pregnant. In fact, it's sensible to let them know as early as you can, so that any necessary plans can be put into place, and your risk assessment (see below) can be carried out. If you're not ready for the rest of your colleagues to know, you can always ask your boss to keep schtum for a while. Let's face it, though, chances are you'll be rumbled early on by some bright spark who's picked up on the fact that you're permanently green around the gills, have virtually set up camp in the toilet, and are no longer the first person standing at the bar come Friday evening.

" Another member of staff was pregnant and 11 weeks ahead of me, so all the attention was on her and I managed to keep it hidden until about 16 weeks. Eventually I had

to use a belt to hold up my suit trousers, as the top fastener wouldn't do up. It felt quite sneaky at the time, but I was reluctant to let people know until after the first scan."
Jenny

When you do come clean about your condition, you need to let your boss know what date your baby is due and when you want your maternity leave and pay to start (see below). You might be required to do this in writing. You'll also need to present them with your maternity certificate (form MATB1), which your midwife will give to you after you're 21 weeks pregnant and which confirms your due date. Your employer must then give you written confirmation of your return date within 28 days (and unless you tell them otherwise, they must assume you're going to take your full maternity leave entitlement of 12 months). You *can* tell your boss if you know for sure you want to come back before the full entitlement period is up (and it's not then set in stone – you can change your mind if you want, as long as you give eight weeks notice of your revised return date).

Many women choose to wait and see how they feel, anyway. Once you've spent some time with your baby you may find you enjoy it so much you want to be at home for longer than you'd originally planned on. Then again, you might realise what an easy life you had before and be champing at the bit to get back to it. Or you may just have done some sums and realised that, financially, you don't have much choice.

" I planned to keep my pregnancy a secret from my boss for a while because other people were leaving at the time and I didn't know how he would react. Between running to the loo all the time and avoiding the pub on a Friday night I was surprised he hadn't noticed. Then the Christmas party came and I had to confess, as I'd run out of excuses."
Marie

Legal rights

What follows is only a basic guide to your legal rights as a pregnant employee. It's a complex subject and one woman's entitlements can differ from another's, depending on a variety of factors. If you've got a helpful human resources manager or well-informed boss who's prepared to take the matter out of your hands, you're in luck. Otherwise, though, you may need to do your homework to make sure your entitlements are being met. As *Modern Girl* Zoe points out: 'My maternity leave started just as the new nine months deal was introduced. I had to inform our human resources department of the change in law as they were a little behind. To be fair, they were very helpful with everything else.'

MATERNITY LEAVE AND PAY

All pregnant employees have the right to take up to 12 months off work – it doesn't matter how long you've worked for a company, or what your hours are. The first 26 weeks of maternity leave is called ordinary maternity leave (OML). You can begin OML up to 11 weeks before your baby is due – the medical view is that eight weeks is a sensible time to take off before your due date, although most women prefer to waddle into work for as long as humanly possible, giving them more time off with their baby once he's born.

> 66 I probably didn't leave work early enough. My daughter was born just 12 days after I started my maternity leave, which really didn't give me time to rest or get ready. 99
> Michelle

If you decide on a leaving date and then change your mind for some reason, you're required to give 28 days notice (although some bosses may be prepared to be more flexible about that). If you have to take time off work because of medical issues related to your pregnancy in the four weeks before your due date, you're automatically considered to have begun your OML. And if you give birth before your planned leave kicks off, your maternity leave will be considered to have started from then on.

You should still be entitled to any contractual benefits you might get (gym membership, for example) during your leave, and your company must continue to make contributions to your pension if they do that already. You're also entitled to take any holiday that builds up in your maternity period – lots of women choose to use this to boost their total amount of maternity leave.

> 66 I ended up going on maternity leave three weeks early, because I was shattered, and my boss was very good about it. I was over-ambitious thinking I could work to 37 weeks. At 34 weeks I'd had enough. I guess you just have to listen to your body and take maternity leave early if you feel you need to – but it's not an easy thing to put a date on, since you're really supposed to make the decision at about 20 weeks, when you're feeling absolutely fine. 99
>
> Nicola

If you were working for an employer when you became pregnant, and you're earning more than £95 a week, you qualify for Statutory Maternity Pay (SMP) which is paid through your employer and (at the time of writing) is 90% of your average pay for the first six weeks, and then £123.06 per week (or 90% of your average earnings if that's less) for a further 33 weeks. So, if you do decide to take the full year's maternity leave you're entitled to, the last three months of your maternity leave will be unpaid.

Some companies have their own maternity pay schemes in place, and you may find that your employer will offer you a more generous rate of maternity pay than the statutory rate. However, this often depends on your having worked there for a certain length of time and is usually on the basis that you'll return to work for a certain period when your maternity leave is over. Bear in mind that if you decide not to go back to work because you want to stay at home with your baby, you may have to pay some of it back.

You may not be entitled to get SMP, for instance if you started your job after becoming pregnant, if you're a casual worker, are self-employed, unemployed, or on a low wage. In these cases, you can usually claim Maternity Allowance instead, which is £123.06 per week for 39 weeks, or 90% of your average pay, whichever is the smaller. This is paid by the government, and you'll need a claim form (MA1) which you can download from the Department of Work and Pensions website.

If you're not sure about what you're entitled to and how to get it, the best source of basic information is the Directgov website.

YOUR PARTNER'S PATERNITY RIGHTS

Your other half may qualify for up to two weeks' paternity leave with statutory paternity pay of £123.06 or 90% of his earnings if that's less – and if he's really lucky, he may even work for a forward-thinking company that offers an enhanced scheme with a better deal than that, perhaps offering full pay for the period. Like you, he'll need to give notice of his intention to take a 'baby break' at least 15 weeks before your due date.

The government introduced a new initiative in 2009, so you can now share your maternity leave with your partner. If you go back to work after 6 months, your partner can stay at home for the next 6 months, to total the 12 months off allowed by law.

TIME OFF FOR ANTENATAL CARE

Your employer must let you have time off for anything that counts as an antenatal care appointment – and this could even include something like a relaxation or parentcraft class, if your midwife or GP has advised you to attend them. If your employer is the suspicious type, they might demand to see an appointment card or a note from a health professional to prove that's really what you're sneaking off for.

'KEEPING IN TOUCH' DAYS

If you're so minded and your employer is keen for you to, you can spend up to 10 days in your workplace, for which you can be paid, during maternity leave. Known as 'keeping in touch' days, these offer a chance for you to keep up with what's going on at work, and maintain links with your colleagues. They don't have to be spent doing your usual job but could involve training or some other special event. Some women find them a useful way of dipping their toes back into their jobs after a long spell away. Keeping in touch days are by no means compulsory though, from either your point of view, or your boss'.

Equally, your employer is entitled to make 'reasonable contact' with you while you're away, if they need to refer to you about a work matter that just can't wait. But they cannot demand you go in to work for any reason – that's down to you.

RETURNING TO WORK AFTER MATERNITY LEAVE

You must give your employer 28 days' notice if you plan to return to work before the end of ordinary maternity leave (in other words, during the first 26 weeks of your year's entitlement), or eight weeks' notice if you plan to go back during additional maternity leave (that is, during the second 26 weeks). If you go back before the ordinary maternity leave period is up, you're entitled to go back to the same job you had before leaving to have your baby. If you go back during your additional maternity leave, you should either get your old job back or be offered something else where the terms and conditions are just as good.

If you decide not to go back to work at all, you have to give your employer whatever notice period your contract demands – it would make sense to do this so that your official leaving date coincides with the end of your maternity leave, to save having to go back for a short period to work out your notice. You won't have to pay back any SMP but if your company has paid you more than the statutory level under enhanced maternity benefits, they could ask you to pay all of it, or some of it, back so you might want to bear that in mind before blowing it all on nursery furnishings. 'It's slightly odd getting maternity pay, since I don't know whether I will go back and I may have to pay them back in a year or less,' admits *Modern Girl* Sarah. 'Obviously the line at work is that I'll be back, so until we decide, we have to take the money – and not spend it!' You may also decide you want to request a return to work with shorter hours or a more flexible set-up.

Requesting flexible working

Lots of women find that returning to work, but on a more flexible or part-time basis than before (either with fewer days, shorter hours, or work-from-home opportunities, perhaps) gives them the work-life balance they're looking for. There's no law that says you *must* be given flexible work if you want it, but anyone who's been with an employer for 26 weeks who has a child under 16 (dads, too) is entitled to request it – and their manager must give it 'serious consideration'. You've nothing to lose by asking.

WHEN YOU'RE THE BOSS

If you run your own company or work for yourself, it will be down to you to decide how long you go on working for and how much time you take off with your baby. You'll probably need to sit down, do some sums, and ask yourself some questions: for example, can you survive on maternity allowance, and if so, for how long? You'll also be responsible for taking care of yourself, and ensuring your own health and safety. Of course, the upside of being your own boss during pregnancy is that if you do really need to spend the morning with your head in a bucket, or switch off your computer and take a nap after lunch, you (usually) can.

" I was so glad to be working from home as I had pelvic girdle pain. I would never have been able to cope with the commute and I'd have had to leave work at around five months. Self-employment makes it much easier to lie on the sofa when you need. "
Antonia

YOUR HEALTH AND SAFETY

By law, your employer must do whatever it takes to protect your health and safety during pregnancy, because if they fail to do so it's automatically considered sex discrimination. Once you've formally notified your employer that you're pregnant, in writing, they must carry out a specific risk assessment based on your individual needs. If any risks are identified you must be informed, and your employer must let you know what they will do to make sure you're not exposed to them. You should make sure they have notice of any medical advice you've been given by a GP or midwife, ideally backed up with a note. Obviously it depends on what your job is, but some potential workplace risks are:

- Lifting or carrying heavy loads.
- Standing or sitting for long periods of time.
- Exposure to infectious diseases; lead; to hazardous chemicals; radioactive material; excessive noise; extremes of temperature; or to shock and vibration.
- Work-related stress.
- Workstations and posture.
- Long working hours.
- Mental and physical fatigue.
- Threat of violence.

If there *is* a risk and your working conditions or hours can't be adjusted to protect you from it, your employer must find you suitable alternative work on the same terms and conditions, and if that can't be done, you should be suspended from work on paid leave, for as long as is necessary. If you're still concerned that your needs aren't being met, do speak up: chat directly to your boss, a human resources manager, or an employee rep, if you have one, and if that doesn't get you anywhere, contact an organisation such as Citizens Advice, ACAS, or the Health and Safety Executive (HSE) for advice.

❝ It was a bit difficult to avoid telling people as I deal with x-ray, chemotherapy and other toxic drugs and I decided early on that my safety was paramount, and sod everyone else. I got the feeling people were thinking, 'you're only pregnant, not ill', but 12-and-a-half hour shifts were a killer towards the end. My midwife was supportive but it was only when I had pains that I gave up, at 33 weeks. Even then I was made to feel like I was 'off sick'. ❞
Zoe

If you need help

In a nutshell, your rights to protection against risks, and for any necessary time off for antenatal care, must be upheld, and you cannot be discriminated against at work simply because you're having a baby. If for some reason you're unhappy with the way you've been treated by your employer, you should seek further advice from a relevant organisation or law company. We've listed some at the back of the book.

Coping with stress

If you do a job where anxiety levels are high, you may quite reasonably worry about the effect it could have on your baby. Fortunately, being fairly resilient little souls, unborn babies will generally weather most of the emotional storms life throws at you – in fact, one recent study found that some moderate, everyday stress could even be *good* for their development.

Severe or prolonged bouts of stress could raise your blood pressure though, and that can cause complications in pregnancy. So if work-related worries are really causing you grief – especially if it's leading to physical problems such as insomnia or headaches – then you might have to gently remind your employer about their legal responsibility to protect your health and safety whilst at work: they have a duty to remove any factors that are causing you stress, where possible, or adjust your conditions or hours accordingly.

If you don't feel you're getting the sympathy you need, chat to your midwife or doctor about it: they might want to sign you off for a while so you can get some rest. (Your boss might not like this – but they will have to lump it.)

Tired all the time?

Plain old exhaustion is one of the hardest things to deal with while working throughout pregnancy, and unfortunately, in most jobs at least, you need to remain in an upright position for the duration of your working day or shift, when in fact what you'd really like to do is lie down and nap. During the first trimester surging hormones can cause an overpowering urge to sleep – and during the third, you might just lose the will to move all together. Both problems are exacerbated if you're having trouble sleeping, which lots of pregnant women do. And naturally, if you do a physical job, or are on your feet for a large part of the day, you'll probably have it even worse.

If you're struggling to get through the day, take a short lunchtime 'power' nap if need be (a snooze of about 15–20 minutes is ideal – any more than that and you may feel worse than when you started). In theory employers have a duty to provide a place for you to rest, if possible, although in reality it may not be practicable. At the very least, a chair and a desk or other surface for you to lay your head down may be better than nothing.

You're likely to find you're fit for nothing but collapsing in a heap on the sofa when you get home after work. As *Modern Girl* Jenny recalls: 'Tiredness in the first trimester was a nightmare, especially as I'd just become deputy head of my primary school. By seven o'clock every evening I was flat out on the settee, comatose.'

Don't make any ambitious plans for weekday evenings if you can help it. Use the time to rest in front of a film, have a soak in the bath, get in some gentle stretches (or maybe even the odd massage from your other half) and get an early night whenever possible.

> **"** My company was signed up for some not-worth-the-paper-it's-written-on 'pregnancy friendly' scheme, which meant a woman from HR came round with a checklist and asked me various questions like: 'Are you working long hours?' to which I replied yes. 'Are you sometimes stressed?' Yes. She said thanks very much, got me to sign her form and I never heard from her again. **"**
> Judy

Be comfortable

Back and pelvic pain are common in pregnancy and can be made worse by sitting or standing for prolonged periods. You also increase your risk of deep vein thrombosis (see page 44) if you sit still for too long, and of dizziness or fainting when you stand. So it's vital to make sure you're as comfortable as you can be while working and that you take regular breaks either to move around or to sit down, as often as necessary. If you're on your feet, wear the most comfortable shoes you can bear – it may not be the look you're hoping for, but your body will thank you for your fashion sacrifice. And if you're on your butt, be sure to take a short break from your workstation for a few moments, preferably at least once or twice an hour.

Make certain your desk and chair are positioned to give you maximum comfort, too – you should ask for a new set-up if your existing one doesn't give you enough space or is causing you discomfort that could otherwise be avoided (see the box below for more tips). And don't forget that your needs may change as your bump gets bigger and sitting becomes increasingly uncomfortable.

Are you sitting comfortably?

- Make sure your chair is high enough. Your feet should be flat on the floor with your hips slightly higher than your knees. Raise your feet if necessary with a box or stool.

- Your computer screen should be positioned directly in front of you.

- Give your spine support with a small cushion placed between the chair and the small of your back.

- Armrests can save the day if you're struggling to hoist yourself out of your chair – if you don't have them, ask your boss to provide.

- Take regular breaks. Get up and move around for a couple of minutes, at least a couple of times an hour.

- Don't cross your legs – it will twist your spine and can affect the circulation. (In fact, get used to sitting like a bloke in the later stages – it's almost impossible to bring your knees together with a very big belly.)

- Sit up straight, but with relaxed shoulders.

- Try to keep your pelvis tilted slightly upwards while you sit.

- You could also aim to fit in some daily ab-strengthening squeezes or pelvic floor exercises (see page 122) while you work.

COPING WITH THE COMMUTE

When you're pregnant, getting to work and back can suddenly seem like the journey from (and to) hell. I took the London Underground daily throughout my first pregnancy, and to this day, I still have the occasional post-trauma flashback. Choice memories include the time I was violently sick on the platform at Waterloo, and a not-so-tactical fainting episode in the ticket queue at Finchley Central. What fun.

Do remember that as part of your rights, your manager needs to ensure you're not getting overtired or overstressed, so if the journey's really getting you down, you could reasonably request a change in start and finish times so you avoid the rush hour, or even, if it's feasible, the chance to work from home on one or more days a week.

Public transport

Getting a seat on public transport is one of the great trials of pregnancy. Ironically, you won't get offered one when you might feel you need it most, in the first trimester, and for most of the second your fellow commuters will probably be so worried that you're simply fat, rather than pregnant, they won't want to ask. Sadly, even being very obviously pregnant is no guarantee that someone will do the decent thing. If no-one's budging, try rubbing your tummy and sighing heavily, while making a show of shifting your weight uncomfortably from one foot to the other. Or just ask outright. A few years ago, London Underground introduced a 'Baby on Board' badge to bluntly alert other passengers to a pregnant woman's presence. You can get one free from London Underground's customer services department, purchase one from eBay for the grand sum of 99p, or, of course, you could make your own.

❝ During my first pregnancy I commuted daily to Central London and it was one of the most stressful things I've ever done. Men In Suits would glance up from their crossword to see me and my huge bump in front of them, then look away quickly so they didn't have to give up their seat. The final straw came when, at 34 weeks, a man got onto a packed bus holding a walking stick and told me to vacate my seat so he could sit down! Everyone pretended not to hear as he swore at me and told me I wasn't disabled so I should get up. Eventually someone gave him a seat, and the next day I told my boss that instead of working until 37 weeks as planned, I was leaving at the end of the week. The stress definitely wasn't worth it — even if the money would have been handy. **"**

Lara

Top tips for commuting

- Leave home a little earlier (or later, if that works better) if it means you can avoid the worst of the rush hour. Even 15 minutes to half-an-hour could make all the difference.

- Once you're showing, unbutton your coat and stick your belly out, so there's no doubt that you're in the family way.

- Be bold. Ask outright for a seat if you feel you need one.

- Wear a 'Baby on Board' badge.

- Don't leave home without a snack and a bottle of water in your bag. You may need sustenance if you feel faint or poorly.

Driving

If you drive to work, make sure you're as comfortable as you can be in the driving seat. If your back hurts, you might get a bit of relief from a small cushion supporting your lower back. Break the journey up to stretch your legs if it's a long one. And once you've got a reasonable-sized bump, consider investing in a 'bump belt', a cushioned strap which can be easily attached, and detached, from your seat belt, keeping it in a position underneath your bump and allowing a safer and more comfortable ride for you and your baby.

FEELING SICK

Whoever coined the term 'morning sickness' obviously hadn't suffered from it since, usually, it goes on all day. Unfortunately, there's very little you can do to ease pregnancy nausea and, as in most cases it's mild (if relentless), you'll have no choice but to soldier on. There's more info and a few other ideas for coping with morning sickness on page 29.

Some managers may be reluctant to make allowances for severe morning sickness (and other pregnancy-related conditions, for that matter). But the law says they cannot discriminate against you in these circumstances – time off for pregnancy-related problems should be considered no different from any general sick leave (except if it happens in the last four weeks before you're due to start your leave, in which case your employer's entitled to clock you off for maternity leave as of then).

If you *do* need to take time off sick because you're ill in pregnancy and you get any grief about it, get a note from your midwife and GP, and stand firm. Remember, you cannot be threatened with discipline or sacking just for taking time off if you're ill through pregnancy. If you are, you could have a good case for an employment tribunal.

You may find that if you're suffering badly from nausea, it's the thing most likely to give you away while you're keeping your pregnancy a secret. Morning sickness in my first pregnancy put paid to my usual breakfast of a bacon butty and large, black coffee, and instead my working day started with a plain white roll and a pint of milk. When, at 13 weeks, I made the official 'announcement' that I was pregnant, my colleagues rolled around laughing for a while before admitting they'd known for only slightly less time than I had.

❝ I was employed as a chef when I found out I was pregnant, and there was no way I could hide it — by six weeks I was throwing up a lot, and just seeing food, let alone working with it in vast quantities, was enough to bring on the vom. So I told my boss, and begged them to just let me go, as I had no intention of going back to work for them and all I could think about was getting out. ❞

Flo

'PREG-HEAD'

There's no conclusive scientific evidence for the existence of 'baby brain', but plenty of the anecdotal variety – ask any woman who's ever been pregnant and she'll no doubt have an example of how her mind went to mush. Theories vary and, in fact, the most recent research on the subject, by a team of experts from Australia, found that cognitive abilities are actually likely to *improve* during pregnancy.

Research aside, though, there's little doubt that, with so much on your mind, exhaustion rampaging through your body, and so many other physical symptoms distracting you, being pregnant can cause many a 'blonde moment', and that can be problematic if you need to keep your mind on whatever your occupation requires of you rather than drifting off into areas more concerned with pain relief, nursery colours, and what on earth you can do to ease the misery of your piles.

'I turned into a complete airhead – my brain ceased to function as normal,' confesses *Modern Girl* Nina. 'I'm usually a very organised and together person, but I'd find myself in board meetings being asked to comment on something and I wouldn't be able to reply. Or I'd turn up for meetings two hours early. Or not at all ...'

There's not a great deal to be done to combat 'preg-head'. Keep a detailed to-do list in front of you at all times – and give yourself a break (literally and figuratively) whenever possible. If you're really struggling, you may need to enlist the sympathy of colleagues by explaining that your brain, as well as your body, has got a lot on right now.

IF YOUR BOSS IS BEING A BUGGER

Some companies are enlightened and experienced in matters of maternity – others aren't. And even if your manager is technically playing the game, you may still be suffering from more resentful attitudes, or a lack of support which can be upsetting. 'My boss was always hard work but he became worse when I was pregnant – everything was my fault,' reveals Marie. 'He knew how to push those buttons and I nearly walked on more than one occasion. I took the matter up with the other partners and the issue was resolved, thankfully.'

If there's no higher level of management you can take the matter to, try to rise above any less-than-helpful mindsets by focusing on doing your job as best you can, thinking about your baby, and reminding yourself that it's a short-term period in your life with an end goal that overrides everything else. Like Marie, make a pledge to yourself that you won't let the bastards get you down. 'There were times when my work was affected by my terrible morning sickness,' she says, 'but I carried on regardless and in my last months I managed to reach a personal best on my commission, which helped pay for lots of the baby essentials.'

Above all, remind yourself that the law is on your side: if you're not happy with the way you're being treated, swot up on your rights and don't be afraid to share that information with your boss, if you need to.

❝ I was allowed to get into work early and leave early to avoid rush hour on the Tube, but that was the only special allowance I got, really. None of the girls I work

with had been through pregnancy so I don't think they really understood how rough I felt, although they did try to be understanding. I'm sure a lot of the time they were complaining about me and to be honest, before I was pregnant myself I might have been guilty of the same.**"**
Jayne

WANT TO GO BACK TO YOUR CAREER?

Although you may not be ready yet to make a decision about what the future holds for you, workwise, it's something to think about. And even if you do have fairly firm ideas at this stage – maybe you know for certain you don't want to go back at all, or maybe you feel very sure that full-time motherhood is definitely not your bag – remember that many women change their minds one way or another once they've dropped their sprog and spent a bit of time with the little critter. Have a general game plan in mind, by all means – but remain open-minded, too.

If you know or think that you're going back to work at some point after your baby's birth, one thing you will need to sort out is some reliable childcare. It's never too early to be looking into this, since popular nurseries and childminders in busy areas often have waiting lists, and you'll need to know about costs if you've got budgeting to do. We've included some useful contact details for organisations concerned with childcare, at the back of the book.

6

Hit and missionary:
your love life during pregnancy

GAGGING FOR IT
OR JUST GAGGING?

" Morning sickness caused the death of my sex drive. It was
rather depressing for my husband to find he had a wife
with a more ample bust, but who had converted overnight
into a bit of a cold fish! Thankfully the second trimester
was fantastic and we had an amazing time enjoying my
new curves and the return of my sex drive. The third

trimester has been a little more quirky as I feel so big and am often full of heartburn!**"**
Sarah

It's what got you into this state in the first place. Yet ironically, sex can become a little scarce in the nine months that follow conception. A very normal experience for women in pregnancy is to have a distinct dearth of bedroom action in the first trimester, as sickness and exhaustion take their toll; a fairly fruity second trimester, as you begin to feel human again and (in some cases) the so-called pregnancy 'horn' takes hold; and a return to the drought during the third, since making love when you're the size of an elephant – and about as flexible – tends to lose appeal. It doesn't always work that way, of course. Some women find their sex drive remains unimpaired through pregnancy. Others are virtually celibate for the duration.

" If my husband kept a sex life diary during both my pregnancies it would read as follows:
'Months 0–3: No chance – the wife is either knackered or vomiting and tells me I smell funny. Months 4–6: God, I'm knackered, I think I'll have to fake a headache tonight. Months 7–9: She says she feels like a beached whale and there's no way I am coming near her. We did try once or twice after she went overdue to get things going. It didn't work and she really wasn't impressed ...**"**
Nina

Why you might not want to have sex when you're pregnant

- You feel too sick.
- You feel too tired.

- You feel fat, and you're self-conscious about it.

- Your piles/back/pelvis/tits/bladder hurt too much (delete as appropriate, or leave all).

- You're worried it could be harmful to your baby.

- You're worried in general. And stressed. And tearful. In short, you're not in the mood.

- You *have* actually got a headache.

- You can't bear the way your other half smells any more.

66 With my first pregnancy I felt very tired and very sick until 13 weeks – and it didn't take long to find out that my husband's 'smell' made me feel even worse! So not only was sex off the cards, cuddling was too. Unfortunately my libido disappeared, I retreated into my own world and managed to come out to remind my husband what sex was like about twice during the whole nine months. Poor bloke!99

Amanda

Pregnancy sex myth busted!

The big 'O' won't bring on premature labour! You may experience mild contractions when you orgasm which can feel a little weird, but they won't be strong enough to trigger labour unless your body's all ready to go in any case.

IS HE HORNY? DO YOU CARE?!

Of course, pregnancy can alter the way men feel about sex, too. It's not unusual for a bloke to be scared, repelled, or just a bit freaked out by the thought because you've got his baby inside you. Some blokes even have a genuine fear of poking the head with their willy. All very well if you're not much in the mood yourself. Rather unfortunate if you happen to be gagging for it.

66 My husband and I slept together once, at 16 weeks, but after that, nothing. He said it was too weird with something inside me. 99

Bev

Pregnancy sex myth busted!

Your partner's penis – however big it may be – will never ever make contact with your baby! The angle of the vagina means that there's no way his willy will bump the baby, unless he has a 90-degree kink in his love tackle. It's anatomically impossible.

Why he may not want to have sex when you're pregnant

- He's also worried it could be harmful to the baby.

- His child is inside you: it's just too weird!

- You're a mother now, or about to be. You've ceased to be a sexual being to him.

- You're not looking your best – in all honesty, he doesn't much fancy you right now.

66 Since sex is meant to bring on labour, and I was late, I ended up having to beg for it. He's a red-blooded male so I got it in the end, but it was strange having to persuade him! I never asked him why this was – I didn't really want to know – but it may be he found me utterly repulsive that size, or he was frightened of hurting the baby. 99

Alex

Pregnancy sex myth busted!

The baby won't get squashed! He's very well cushioned in his amniotic sac, and will be completely untroubled by your bedroom antics.

---

66 To be honest I haven't found it any different when pregnant, just less appealing when coming near the end of pregnancy because I am so uncomfortable and tired. 99

Sara

MAKE SEX WORK

Sex in pregnancy can be a good thing, so if you *can* keep up something resembling a sex life for at least some of the nine months, there are lots of benefits to be had. For instance:

- There's no need to fumble for a condom or fret that you forgot your pill that morning.
- Increased blood flow to the pelvic region can mean faster, bigger and better orgasms.
- Your boobs may be a growing attraction.

- It will make you feel emotionally close to each other.

- You don't have much choice but to experiment with sexual positions.

- It's a good way to exercise your pelvic muscles, so excellent preparation for birth.

- It's sex purely for the heck of it (which could be relevant if you had fertility issues before, and were more concerned with making a baby than making love).

- It will make you feel relaxed and sleepy – the perfect antidote to stress and insomnia.

- It might just help move things along if you're due or overdue.

- Once the baby's born you probably won't make love for ages. In other words, *get some now, while you still can…!*

Pregnancy sex myth busted!

Having sex won't cause you to have a miscarriage! Although, if you've had one before or you've had some bleeding, your doctor or midwife might advise you to abstain, just to be on the safe side.

The pregnancy horn

Higher levels of hormones and an increased blood flow in the pelvic area mean it all becomes a bit swollen and super-sensitive down there and thus – in theory – faster arousal and better, longer orgasms. (Presumably this is Mother Nature's little apology for the host of horrors she's inflicted elsewhere on your body.) However, it has to be said that plenty of women don't experience any more stirrings down below than is normal – I know I didn't, sadly.

❝ The truth: I just couldn't have been less interested! I either felt sick or knackered or just plain old fat and

unattractive. All this business about feeling extra sexy seems to have totally passed me by."
Rebecca

There's also a flipside to this particular pregnancy 'perk': the area can become too sensitive, making arousal and orgasm uncomfortable. Boobs, too, can be affected by a hormonal blood rush, and may feel unbearably sore.

" I absolutely loved sex during pregnancy and couldn't get enough of it. Being a bit skinny I loved my changing shape and felt positively voluptuous. Just two hours before going into labour with my eldest, my exhausted husband was to be heard groaning and saying, 'Oh God, not again'."
Mandy

Oral sex

Making love doesn't have to mean penetration and even if you don't fancy full-on sex, you don't have to give up on intimacy. You could still have quite a lot fun with some good, old-fashioned mutual masturbation, and oral sex doesn't take much effort – especially if it's him on you. One thing might affect this, though: hormonal influences can make your vaginal secretions heavier than usual, and they could smell and taste a bit different. Of course, there's no particular reason why you can't return the favour – except perhaps if you feel sick, have a funny taste in your mouth, can't abide the smell of just about anything, or cannot actually bend over because your back hurts or your belly's getting in the way … Don't feel under pressure to dole out blow jobs just because you feel bad about enforcing a sex drought on the poor man. He'll survive.

Pregnancy sex myth busted!

Cunnilingus will not kill you! Boy-on-girl oral sex is perfectly safe. However, just in case he was considering it, don't let your partner blow hard inside you. There's a small risk, in theory, that it could cause an air bubble to enter your circulatory system and lead to a potentially fatal embolism.

Other ways of being intimate

Of course, you don't even have to get sexy to get intimate. A massage, or a simple naked cuddle can feel pretty good and will help remind you that you're a couple, and not just two people sharing a bed who are about to have a baby together.

Finding a comfortable position

Straightforward missionary ceases to become a comfortable option once you've got a significant belly on you – not only will it get in the way, but lying flat on your back can put pressure on the main vein, and that can cause dizziness. A pillow under your bottom should raise your lower back enough to prevent this, and if you position yourself right on the edge of the bed, and get your man to do his duty standing (or kneeling) up, you'll be sorted.

Woman-on-top isn't a bad alternative, either, although it does mean you've got to do the work which isn't ideal if you're tired, and he'll have a serious eyeful of your belly, which you may feel self-conscious about or he might not like. For variation, you could try this sitting on a chair (make sure it's a strong one).

Best of all is probably anything with a behind-entry theme: 'doggy style' with you on your hands and knees can work well. If that doesn't appeal there's the gentler version, 'spoons', where you lie down together on your sides facing the same way with him behind you.

You'll have to use your imaginations a bit when it comes to sex in late pregnancy – chances are you'll try out more positions during pregnancy than you did in your first three months together. A sense of humour, and a selection of pillows, may help.

Pregnancy sex myth busted!

The baby won't be exposed to an infection! The thick mucus plug which seals off the cervix means bacteria can't get through, and your baby is perfectly safe.

Keep talking

It's totally normal for one or both halves of a couple to go off sex for some reason during pregnancy, and that's fine. Any half-decent partner – however sex-starved – should be able to see it as a temporary phase in the context of your whole lives together (the fact that there might not be much sex around for a while after you've had the baby is neither here nor there. Sex lives do tend to get put on hold when you become parents, and fortunately, they almost always come back again.)

If things are lacking in the bedroom department, it's a really good idea to talk about why, if you can, and to make sure that there are plenty of kisses, cuddles and touching to make up for it. It's all too easy to feel rejected when your partner doesn't want sex with you, even if they do have a damn good excuse for not being much in the mood, so it's important to make sure the 'unwilling' party lets the other one know they still care.

❝ I've never felt less sexy, less glamorous, less horny or less up for it than when pregnant. Pity my poor, extremely

155

patient and understanding husband, who didn't get much, ahem, relief at all during the whole nine months. **"**
Lara

BRINGING ON LABOUR

It's a well-worn piece of advice that making love when your baby is due is a good way to kickstart proceedings. There is some scientific basis for this, which is probably why most expectant couples give it at least one shot in the closing weeks (when in fact, for many women, sex is the least important thing on their minds). The hormone oxytocin is released during orgasm, which makes the womb contract and helps to 'limber' up the cervix ready for its big role in birth. Added to that, semen contains prostaglandin, a hormone-like substance which is said to soften the cervix. Prolonged bouts of nipple fondling can also encourage a release of oxytocin – however you do have to fondle them for quite long periods if this really is going to work (see page 216). And why ever not?

You shouldn't have sex if your waters have broken or leaking, or if you've had a 'show' (see page 214), which means the mucus plug sealing your cervix has come away, or partly come away, as it could leave your baby vulnerable to infection.

" Our sex life was non-existent mainly due to sickness, but it did pick up near the end of my pregnancy – especially right at the end when trying to induce labour. (It worked!)**"**
Jane

Pregnancy sex myth busted!

The baby has no idea you are shagging! He might have an idea something exciting's afoot because your heartbeat's all over the place – and he'll hear you, if you've a tendency to be 'vocal' about these things. And yes, he might even decide to get in on the act by kicking and moving around a bit. But he doesn't know you're at it. Really.

WHEN NOT TO HAVE SEX

Your doctor or midwife might suggest you give sex a miss during one or more parts of your pregnancy if they reckon it could be risky: for instance, if you've a history of miscarriage, have suffered bleeding, your waters have burst early, or have leaked (in case of infection), or if you have or could have placenta praevia (see page 17). Hold off sex until you've spoken to your midwife if you do experience any amount of bleeding – although it may be due to something harmless such as cervical erosion (see page 66), it should always be investigated.

Some sexually transmitted diseases, such as genital herpes, syphillis, gonorrhoea, or chlamydia, could infect your baby either in the womb or during delivery, and prove seriously harmful to him. If you suspect you're carrying one of these, or that your partner is, let your midwife or doctor know straight away so they can arrange for testing and treatment.

66 Sex, what's sex?! We're not allowed to have any for the first 14 weeks because of my history of fertility problems and miscarriage. No fun at all! It's then quite nerve-racking getting back into things after such a long break. 99

Sara

LOOKING AFTER YOUR RELATIONSHIP

It's not just the physical side of your love life that's affected by pregnancy. It can be a challenging time emotionally, too. You may have numerous symptoms to cope with – none of which he can do anything about, or have any inkling of the extent of their awfulness – and unpredictable mood swings that you must both contend with.

The upshot of that may well be large doses of resentment. 'I was furious that my life had changed so so much and his hadn't,' confesses *Modern Girl* Rebecca. 'Furious that my body was getting trashed, and his wasn't. That he could sleep, and I couldn't. That he could still drink and indulge, and I couldn't. I hated being pregnant, and he just couldn't empathise. And he wasn't the least bit interested in reading any of the books!'

66 I think the tiredness of pregnancy put a real downer on our relationship, and you know how tiredness works — you just get emotional and grumpy over nothing, and end up going to bed feeling rotten about everything. In fact, we got at each other so much during the first half (as well as the first few weeks of having a baby), we're not certain we want another one. **99**
Jill

While you seethe, he's probably feeling frustrated, since his attempts to help are fruitless (and, more than likely, extremely ungratefully received). On top of all that, both of you are likely to be anxious and scared about whether your baby will be OK, the birth, and the huge responsibility that lies ahead as parents. And he could well be feeling the pressure – with a child to provide for and a partner who may not be earning the full whack for a while – of being the main breadwinner. Add in the fact that your sex life may not be going with a swing any more, and you can see why pregnancy can put a strain on even the strongest of relationships. The best thing you can do to keep your love for each other ticking over healthily during pregnancy is to talk to each other.

> **66** There may have been a few 'hormonal' moments when I lost the plot with him, but I think I can honestly say we were closer during pregnancy. It helped that he loved my changing body and my ever-growing bump – well, that's what he said, anyway!**99**
> Lara

Silence can breed resentment, so try to let him know (preferably in a calm and measured way, rather than screaming at him) how you're feeling. Although he will never truly know what hell you are going through in order to bring his child into the world, you can make sure he's got some idea by thrusting an informative guide such as this one in his hand.

Talking's a two-way street of course, so make sure you extend an ear to his woes, too. If you're arguing more than is usual, be sure to kiss and make up before things get out of hand. And pencil in as many slots as possible to spend with each other: even if time's tight because you're both working and spare moments are devoted to sorting the house out, shopping for the baby, and trying to get a bit of rest in, make a date with each other one of your main priorities. Discuss your plans for the birth, and for parenthood, and talk about the changing phases of your pregnancy by all means. But sometimes it's a good idea to put the whole pregnancy/baby thing out of the equation for a while, (your huge bump notwithstanding), and talk about something completely different.

Try, too, to give each other a bit of space where necessary. You may not be out with friends as much as you once were because you're not feeling very sociable, but keep up your old friendships and aim to spend time with people other than your other half – and encourage him to do his own thing, too. A little absence can, as they say, make the heart grow fonder – and will also stop you getting under each other's feet.

Above all, try to keep in mind that pregnancy is a temporary phase in any couple's shared lifetime. Happily, most people find that ultimately, pregnancy and parenthood brings them closer, not further apart.

❝ His nurturing side has come to light, and he's so excited, he's like a kid at Christmas, which is sweet and encouraging. It's nice to feel special, protected and cared for — even if at times he's a touch neurotic!**❞**
Claire

Any problems you're up against now will usually fade into insignificance once your baby's born and it becomes clear that what you've been through was a means to a wonderful end. (Of course, having a new baby can put also put all sorts of pressures on a couple's love life – but that's another subject.)

If your relationship really seems in trouble, it would be a good idea to thrash things out before the baby's arrival. You might want to consider some couples counselling, through an organisation like Relate. There are some useful addresses at the back of the book.

❝ Pregnancy puts your love on a deeper level. When he's shaved your legs for you because you can't reach, put up with huge mood swings, agreed to eat his chips in another room because you can't stand the smell of vinegar, and made love to you when you look and feel like a beached whale, then you know you've got a good man.**❞**
Sara

7

Delivery schedule: making plans for your baby's arrival

Unless you're in total denial, you'll want to give plenty of advance thought to the momentous event that comes right at the end of pregnancy. Birth can be a pretty nerve-racking prospect, especially when it's your first baby and you don't have much else apart from other people's birth stories, and horrible scenes from *Casualty,* to go by. But one thing's certain: this baby's coming out of you, and you need to be prepared for it.

While you can never really know what birth's like until you've actually been through it, you can help yourself be ready for it by doing your 'homework' (reading this book will be a good start). You might even be able to influence how yours turns out by making some tentative plans.

The important thing is to bear in mind is that where birth's concerned – particularly your first – nothing's guaranteed. So when it comes to planning yours, you should keep an open mind until the time comes.

WHERE YOU'RE GOING TO HAVE YOUR BABY

There are three basic options when it comes to where you're going to give birth:

- Consultant-led hospital unit.

- Midwife-led (or GP-led) unit.

- Home birth.

As this is a pretty important decision and could have quite a big impact on how your birth turns out, you'd be wise to give it some thought. What follows is a broad outline, but there's lots more detail at BirthChoiceUK: an impartial website offering loads of information on the choices you need to make, and what's available in your area.

Once you've made a decision about where to give birth, you don't have to stick to it. You're entitled to change your mind at any point.

CONSULTANT-LED HOSPITAL UNIT

The majority of women choose a consultant-led hospital maternity unit. And although there's no doubt that some can seem a bit grim, decorated as they often are with peeling paint, and furnished with a selection of scary-looking items of equipment, they do offer the reassurance of access to the whole gamut of pain relief options, and any medical aids that may be required. There'll always be an obstetrician on call if needed during the pregnancy or birth, and you'll be in the best place should an emergency arise. All of which is probably why, for the vast majority of mums, a hospital maternity unit seems the most appealing place to have your baby the first time round.

If your nearest hospital is truly grotty, bear in mind that you're entitled to choose another, even if it's not in your area. However, for obvious reasons, it makes sense to go for one you can get to fairly swiftly if necessary. (Always better to give birth inside a building, than by the side of the road.)

Once you're booked in, you'll generally be offered a chance to take a look round the maternity unit. While this can be reassuring and informative, it may also leave you feeling a bit wobbly – just like *Modern Girl* Isla. 'I visited the hospital at 25 weeks,' she says. 'There were bars on the side of the bed and it felt like I was walking on to the set of *One Flew Over The Cuckoo's Nest*. I cried because I really didn't want to have my baby there. Luckily the same hospital had a gorgeous birthing unit downstairs, with a pool, and I decided go there instead.'

66 My hospital tour and antenatal classes were cancelled (good old NHS), so I didn't visit the hospital beforehand, but I don't think that mattered a bit. 99
Flo

If you do visit your chosen maternity ward, use it as a chance to ask questions and familiarise yourself with basic stuff like where the loos and nearest catering facilities are – let's face it, when the time comes to check in for real, you'll have other stuff on your mind. You can also find out what potentially useful equipment there is available: for instance, a birthing pool, aids such as birthing balls, comfy cushions, or bean bags, and a CD or cassette player. Delivery rooms these days tend to be more comfortable and better equipped for birth than they used to be. But if not, you might be able to bring what you need with you.

66 We did the hospital tour but unfortunately all it did was freak me out when I suddenly realised that I was actually going to have to give birth. It was useful for my husband, though – at least he knew where the loos and the vending machines were. 99
Lara

MIDWIFE-LED UNIT

In some areas, and providing you're not at high risk of some complication arising during birth, you may also be offered the option of having your baby in the more 'homely' setting of a midwife-led maternity unit, sometimes called a GP-led unit, or a birthing centre, and often described as providing a sort of 'halfway house' between a hospital and a home birth. These usually operate independently, but some are attached to hospitals. There are growing numbers of these sorts of units, but still, not every area has one yet so you may find that you just don't have the option for geographical reasons.

Because they're staffed by midwives, you won't see any scary looking forceps-wielding consultants in green coats in a birthing centre. The focus is more likely to be on a relaxed and natural experience, and it certainly seems to pan out that way in most cases – statistics show that women who have their babies in this kind of unit are less likely to go on to need assistance in the form of vacuum extraction (ventouse) or forceps (see page 232), or to go on to have a caesarean section (see page 184 and page 234).

Birthing centres are equipped with the things that make natural birth more of a possibility – water pools, for example – and are likely to be more comfortable all round. There may also be room for your other half to stay in there with you. But there won't be an obstetrician or anaesthetist immediately to hand which means you won't get an epidural here (a fact that you could regret bitterly when you realise just how effing painful your natural birth has turned out to be, after all), and there are no facilities for surgery, or for special baby care. And of course, in the event of certain emergencies, you'd still face the inconvenience of being transferred by ambulance to the nearest appropriate hospital – although, in some cases, that will be right next door, which is reassuring.

❝ The Edgware Birth Centre was a dream of a place, where they make you so welcome and relaxed and approach the whole birth as if it's something completely natural.

I prayed I would be low risk so I would be OK to have my baby there.**"**
Marie

HOME BIRTH

If you're very hospital-averse, or simply a plucky soul who's determined to do the whole darn thing as nature intended, risks and all, you might want to consider giving birth in the comfort and privacy of your own home. I would never knock this option, as I can see that when things do go right, your own home would certainly be the perfect place to have your baby. Indeed, I know plenty of *Modern Girls* who've popped one out in their lounge only to be tucked up half-an-hour later under their own duvet. Needless to say, they then tend to wax lyrical about how joyful it all was. You will also be under the care of just one or two community midwives who'll stick with you throughout the whole experience, rather than subject to the changing shift patterns of the average maternity unit.

But there's absolutely no doubt about the drawbacks of this option: if anything happens that's beyond the capabilities of the midwife who's with you to cope with, you'll be bundled in an ambulance faster than you can say 'epidural', and whisked to your nearest hospital anyway, blue lights ablaze. Not only that, but you won't have anything more than gas and air (see page 173) at your disposal for pain relief (although some midwives will administer pethidine, see page 175). As you'll see later in more detail, giving birth is really bloody painful indeed – and when it's your first, it's often prolonged, which means you can start off coping OK with the contractions but, 24 hours later, find that biting your lip and breathing is no longer enough for you.

All of which is no doubt why it's still a fairly unusual experience, with an average one in 50 babies in the UK born at home. I can say with certainty that a home birth wouldn't have been a good option for me

– following both my births I had a retained placenta (see page 232) which I needed surgery to remove (not to mention the first-time-round epidural, for which I recall weeping like a baby whilst still a mere 3cm dilated.

All that said, if a woman wants to have her baby at home and there are no obvious major risks involved, then she should certainly be able to. In theory, the choice is open to all women, although in reality, there are still some of areas where you might be discouraged, or even told outright it won't be possible, with staff shortages or cutbacks usually given the blame.

And wherever you live, you're likely to be discouraged from having a home birth if there's any complicating factor that means you'd be safer giving birth in a hospital: for instance, if you have a medical condition like pre-eclampsia, if you're expecting twins, or if your baby's in the breech position as you come close to your due date. Some health professionals are even pretty categoric in their belief that home birth isn't a sensible option for *any* woman giving birth for the first time.

Pro-homebirthers are pretty vocal in their opposition to this sort of attitude. They point out that it's no more dangerous for low-risk women, even first-timers, to give birth at home than at hospital.

Do have a good read up on the subject if home birth is something you'd like to look into (I've included some sympathetic sources of info in the appendix). And if you want to go for it, go for it.

> 66 When I told my midwife I was considering a home birth she told me she didn't think it was a good idea. I persevered, and was told to go away and make a decision – without being given any information to actually base one on! Thankfully I managed to speak to another, lovely midwife, who was much more enthusiastic. 99
>
> Judy

Some homebirthers opt to hire an independent midwife so they can get comprehensive support. This is a pretty expensive option (fees range from £1,500 to £4,000), but women who have done so usually report high levels of satisfaction. There's more information on the website of the Independent Midwives Association. There are also a number of organisations, support groups and websites which are included at the back of the book.

66 I had no opposition at all to my home birth. It depends on the area you live in as to how pro or anti the staff generally are and I'm lucky to be in a pro-home-birth area. 99
Kelly

MAKING A BIRTH PLAN

Once you know where you're having your baby, it's a good idea to make some more specific plans for the sort of birth you want, or rather, that you hope for. Things to think about include pain relief, birthing positions, and stuff that you might prefer to avoid, *if possible*. What isn't a good idea is having a rigid idea of how you want things to pan out because, ultimately, you don't know what fate has in store for you on the day and how you'll cope with it, anyway. So plan by all means, but don't imagine those plans to be set in stone. Promise yourself you'll see what happens when the time comes.

Many people would argue that 'making a birth plan' is as futile a use of a pregnant woman's time as shopping for stilettos: you simply cannot 'plan' what's going to happen during your labour. But still, there's no harm in considering your utopia. If you do have any feelings one way or another about how – in an ideal world – you'd like your baby's birth to go, it's worth getting it down on paper. At the very least, it will help you confront the issues that are likely to arise.

During labour, assuming there's time, your midwife should be happy to take a look at yours and to do what she can to abide by your wishes as far as is possible. On the other hand, there's always the possibility that it never makes it out of the bag …

66 Birth plans? I think they're bollocks, frankly. How can you have firm ideas about one of the most intense experiences of your life, something totally different to anything you've ever experienced before?99
Shona

Above all, remember this: if you do make a birth plan, there's no point in making any inflexible pledges or demands, because you just don't know what's going to happen and how you'll cope. Avoid statements like, 'I absolutely refuse to have this baby taken out of me surgically', for example, or, 'Strap me to the bed and inject the epidural on my arrival'. Instead, stick to phrases like, 'I hope to avoid a delivery by ventouse or forceps and would like to be given time to consider measures such as these if considered necessary.' And do cover all eventualities, if you can. When I wrote mine the first time, I was canny enough to predict that I'd be begging for an epidural before too long and made sure I mentioned it in the plan, just in case I was rendered incoherent with pain and unable to ask for one. Quite rightly, as it turned out.

If you're not sure what to put in your birth plan, there are some ideas below. You'll also find some good advice on the NHS Choices website. Some maternity units even provide a printed form to help you get your plan on paper. Make sure it's typed or written neatly, so that the midwife can actually make sense of it. And do make your birth plan in cahoots with your antenatal care team. They'll be able to let you know if there's anything about your personal circumstances that might be relevant.

66 I wrote a birth plan. It was quite long, but it was essentially summed up in the last sentence – 'I will consider whatever is necessary and go with the flow! 99
Amanda

What you might want to include if you make a birth plan

- The sort of pain relief you think you want – and any that you'd quite like to avoid.

- Who your birth partner's going to be.

- What sort of positions you're keen to try out – for instance, if you think you'd prefer to be standing or kneeling to have your baby and whether you'd like to remain active if possible.

- Whether you'd like to give the birthing pool a whirl, if they have one.

- Any desire you may have to avoid certain procedures – induction, or an episiotomy, for example – if at all possible.

- If one method of intervention is preferable to you over another – for instance, if you think a vacuum extraction delivery would be less of a concern than one involving forceps.

- Whether or not you're happy to have an injection to speed up the delivery of the placenta.

- If your partner is keen to cut the umbilical cord.

- How you plan to feed your baby. If you want to breastfeed, the midwife will probably help you to try straight away.

Of course, for many women, a birth plan may amount to nothing more than the following phrase: 'I am happy for you to do whatever it takes to help me give birth to my baby safely'. And that's an eminently sensible view.

> " I didn't bother with a birth plan because although I wanted to avoid any intervention, at the end of the day all I wanted was a healthy baby and if that meant cutting me open, then I would have said do it. "
> Nicola

HOPING FOR A 'NATURAL BIRTH'?

You might hear or read an awful lot of stuff about 'natural' or 'normal' birth during your pregnancy. Definitions of natural birth vary, but it basically means going through labour and delivery without intervention or pain relief (other than stuff like massage, water, or breathing techniques – and gas and air's usually considered allowable too, under 'natural birth' rules).

Certainly there are potential advantages to a natural birth: research suggests if you're one of the minority who have one, you're more likely to have less postnatal pain and a faster recovery. Some people say that it's a more rewarding way to have a baby, which means you're more likely to look back on your birth with a sense of achievement. And some say it makes for easier bonding with your child, and more chance of successful breastfeeding.

> " I planned to the nth degree, down to what music I wanted played, for a natural birth. Absolutely all of it was utterly useless and none of it came to fruition – the water birth and calmness went out of the window in an induction/forceps nightmare. "
> Sheridan

Natural birth is an emotive issue. Many people believe that, if women were left to their own devices with the help of a supportive midwife and without threat from c-section obsessed doctors, far more births could be natural than are, and far less intervention could be carried out than is. These people may well be right. But the truth is you're often too bewildered, too scared, or too exhausted to do anything other than put your faith in whichever professionals are around at the time. And it may well be that all you really care about, at that point, is for your baby to be born in one piece and for your experiences in the delivery room to be over.

Do by all means plan for a natural birth if it's something that's important to you. But don't bank on it. And don't think for a minute you'll somehow have a less than ideal birth experience if it turns out not to be a 'natural' one. The truth is that sometimes – often, in fact – it's *just not possible* to have a natural birth. So it's best not to get too hung up on the idea.

> 66 I felt very determined to have a natural water birth with no internal examinations or drugs, and that's what I got. I think it's important to decide what kind of birth you want and to be assertive in achieving it. I was so glad I wasn't all woozy with drugs, so I could feel it fully. 99
> Marie

What you can do to improve your chances

- Research having a home birth, or going to a midwife-led birthing centre. Having your baby in hospital doesn't mean you automatically forgo your chances of a natural birth (although statistically, it does reduce your chances). Make it clear that's what you'd like in your birth plan – and make sure your birth partner's fully briefed so they can pipe up during labour.

- Sign up for NCT antenatal classes, where the focus is usually biased in favour of natural or low-intervention birth, and you can learn breathing and relaxation techniques. You could also look into alternative private antenatal courses such as active birth classes or antenatal yoga.

- Consider a water birth. Research has shown that women who spend part of their labour in a birthing pool are less likely to go on to have pain relief such as pethidine, or an epidural, and there's also evidence that it can reduce the likelihood of tearing or needing an episiotomy. Some women use water in the first stage only, for pain relief, getting out to actually deliver their baby. But others choose to actually have their baby in the pool. Although a particularly popular option during a home or birthing centre delivery, many hospital maternity units are also equipped with a birthing pool these days. However, they may have fairly strict guidelines about who they'll let in. There's more about water as a method of pain relief on page 178.

- Look into alternative methods of pain relief and relaxation such as hypnotherapy, acupuncture, aromatherapy, massage, and breathing techniques (see p 180).

- Choose another woman as your birth partner. Research shows that having a female companion in the delivery room with you improves your likelihood of having a birth without intervention.

- If he's not there already, encourage your baby into the right position prior to birth (see page 210).

- Prepare for 'natural' birth positions such as standing up or kneeling. You'll be more confident about using them during the birth itself if you've tried them out beforehand, so aim to get in some practice.

PAIN RELIEF OPTIONS

Having a baby hurts. Quite how much it hurts, how long it will hurt for, and how you personally cope with the pain are all factors that it's impossible to generalise about. And although I would like to be able to give you a full and detailed explanation of the levels of pain I myself experienced during my two labours, I can't, very well. I've kind of blocked it out.

Fortunately for modern women, medical science now offers us a number of pain relief options. A minority of women make it through birth without, either through choice or because circumstances dictate (if your baby comes in a hurry and there just isn't time, for example). But in the vast majority of births, pain relief of some kind is used.

Do your research and have a good, hard think about the type of pain relief you think will be right for you, and which if any you're fairly certain you won't want (for instance, some women rule out an epidural early on because of a fear of big needles). And by all means write it down in your birth plan, if you want. But whatever you decide, be totally and utterly prepared to change your mind (or to have it changed for you) when the time comes. You just cannot predict how intense, how prolonged, and how bearable the pain is going to be.

Entonox – gas and air

What is it?

Gas and air, a mix of 50% oxygen and 50% nitrous oxide, is administered through a mouthpiece or mask from which you breathe it in. It's readily accessible and you're in control – chances are that when no-one's looking, your birth partner will demand a toke, too.

When can I have some?

Any time during labour and birth, and whenever you feel the need. Since it also comes in portable canisters, it's one of the few forms of pain relief you can rely on if you're giving birth at home. You'll also be able to use it if you're giving birth in water, unlike most other forms of pain relief.

Is it any good?

It's one of the least powerful forms of pain relief for birth, but it can certainly take the edge off, so it's a good option in the earlier phases before the going gets tough. As it can take up to a minute for the effects to kick in, it's best to take it when you feel a contraction coming, rather than right in the middle of one.

Are there any drawbacks?

Gas and air creates a sort of 'high' which can render you woozy, like being really drunk – a sensation that might make you feel a bit out of control. It can also lead to a dry mouth and can sometimes make you feel nauseous. Otherwise it has no adverse effects and is safe for you and your baby.

> ❝ My first labour was just three hours from the first contraction and I got through it with just gas and air. I'd hoped it would be enough, but believe me I'm no martyr and I had the epidural as an option on my birth plan – just lucky I didn't need one. ❞
> Sara

TENS machine

What is it?

A TENS (Transcutaneous Electrical Nerve Stimulation) machine is a little box which emits electrical pulses through four wires and four sticky pads, which you fix to your back. It works by intercepting pain signals to your brain, and by stimulating the release of endorphins; the body's natural pain-busting hormones. They have dials with which you can control the frequency and intensity of the pulses – start off low and increase them as the contractions get stronger.

When can I have some?

As early as you like – as it takes up to an hour for your body to respond you should make sure you get it on in good time. You'll probably want to take it off towards the later stages of labour, as it's unlikely to help with very strong contractions and all the wires will just be a nuisance. You'll need some help from your birth partner or midwife to stick the pads on in the right place. You can't use a TENS machine in a birthing pool. Electric shocks and all that.

Is it any good?

Opinions vary – some women find them helpful, others say they're not particularly effective.

What are the drawbacks?

I turned the voltage up too high by mistake on mine, causing a pulse so strong it made me squeal. You won't be able to get a back massage, either, as the pads will get in the way. TENS machines aren't routinely available in maternity units – although some NHS trusts lend them out – so if you want one you'll probably need to buy or hire it. They're available from a whole range of places, including specialist companies and from big shops such as Boots or Mothercare. Expect to pay between £20 and £30 to hire, and around £50–£60 to buy.

66 I used a TENS machine, which was excellent, and gas and air, which was a waste of time but gave me something to do. 99

Nina

Painkilling drugs such as pethidine, meptid, and diamorphine

What is it?

These painkilling drugs (also known as analgesics) are usually given via an injection in the thigh or bum, or occasionally direct into the bloodstream, through a fine tube inserted into a vein in your arm. Midwives are able to administer them, so there'll be no need to call in a doctor if you want some. You may also be able to take control of your own dosage if the unit has a PCA (Patient Controlled Analgesia) device. Pethidine is the most widely used, while meptid and diamorphine are only available in some units. Check in advance what's available in yours.

When can I have it?

You can have any of these at any point, except when you're coming close to the pushing stage, as they're more likely to have a harmful effect on your baby if given too late in labour. You may be able to have pethidine at a home birth, but many midwives are reluctant to administer it because of the risks to the baby.

Is it any good?

Reports from women vary – some say they were effective, others that they were little or no help in relieving the pain, although they usually make it easier to rest and relax between contractions.

What are the drawbacks?

They can make you feel very drowsy, dizzy, or sick. If too much is given, or they're given too late, these sort of drugs can hang around in your baby's system for several days after the birth, which could slow down his breathing and cause him to be very sleepy, perhaps affecting his feeding.

66 I hadn't wanted pethidine, but my other half persuaded me it would be fine and that it would help to relax me, and it did. 99

Jane

Epidural

What is it?

An anaesthetic injection into the spine, which numbs the nerve supply that serves the uterus and cervix giving complete, and fast, relief from pain. Although quite a lot of women say they'd rather avoid one when planning a first birth, quite lot also end up having one: around a quarter. Some hospitals offer a mobile epidural – this is a lower dose injection which gives pain relief without taking away all feeling in the legs, so you can still move around.

When can I have some?

As soon as the pains start to become intolerable. The effects last for several hours, but you may need 'top-up' doses. However, it's best if it's worn off by the time you come to start pushing, as you'll be able to do so much more effectively if you've got sensation down there. Epidurals have to be administered by an anaesthetist, so you may have to wait if he or she is busy elsewhere in the hospital – women have been known to wait so long that it's too late. In some hospitals, you might not get one at all if it's the middle of the night. You won't be able to have one at home, or in a birthing centre.

Is it any good?

Very effective indeed, usually – in theory, you shouldn't feel a thing once it's kicked in.

What are the drawbacks?

You can end up numb to your toes, and that means you can't get up and walk around. An epidural can weaken contractions and the lack of sensation can make it harder to push, so you're more likely to need a forceps or ventouse delivery (see below). You'll need a drip in your arm, as a precaution in case your blood pressure drops and you need to be given fluid urgently, and your baby will also need to be continuously monitored. You're likely to have a catheter too (a tube going into your bladder, to remove wee), as you can't feel whether your bladder is full or not, all of which means your mobility will be restricted. Sometimes there can be side effects, such as a fever, shaking, headache, or backache.

66 I'd say go with an epidural every time! Don't understand why you wouldn't. 99
Coral

ALTERNATIVE METHODS OF PAIN RELIEF

You don't have to be a kaftan-wearing type to take a look at natural, alternative methods of pain relief. Lots of midwives acknowledge – and even practise – these techniques these days, so if you decide to 'go alternative' in the delivery room, you might find you've got support.

The jury's out on just how much these treatments can help and, if they do at all, how they work. However the fact remains that lots of women find one – or several, used in conjunction – helpful in the early stages of labour. And a small number will even manage to get through the whole thing on nothing more than positive thought and a back rub.

Just don't pin your hopes too firmly on an alternative method of pain relief. Keep an open mind – you may think aromatherapy massage will see you through 24 hours of hard labour and find when you get to it, that only an epidural will do.

Water

Sinking into a birthing pool full of warm water is widely reported to be a very effective method of natural pain relief. It's available now in many maternity units and is becoming an increasingly popular choice. Women who've used it with success say that water can aid comfort and relaxation, and often claim it helped them towards a 'calm' and 'peaceful' experience. However, once in the water, you won't be able to have any other pain relief apart from gas and air – you'll have to get out if you want something stronger.

❝ I was totally prepared to take all pain relief offered and didn't rule anything out. As it turned out I was lucky. I went in the pool and didn't need more than the water, and gas and air.**❞**
Rebecca

Acupuncture

This ancient Chinese therapy involves the insertion of fine needles into various points of the body, which, it's said, stimulates the energy channels and releases endorphins, the body's natural painkilling hormones. As with most alternative therapies, there's no real scientific evidence in its favour, and many doctors are sceptical. If you decide it could be for you, find a qualified private practitioner through the British Acupuncture Council.

Aromatherapy

Based around the power of a multitude of different natural 'essential' oils, aromatherapy is supposed to have wide-ranging, positive effects on the mind and body. These oils can be administered in a variety of ways, for example with massage, or through inhalation from a burner or vaporiser, or drops of oil infused on a hankie. Some oils are more suitable than others for labour, so do consult a trained aromatherapist for advice – or at least do some careful homework. It's unlikely that aromatherapy in itself will do very much to boost your pain threshold. But it may well aid relaxation and therefore help you cope better in the early part of labour – and it might just take the edge off the unpleasant hospital smell in the delivery room. (Essential oils shouldn't be put directly in the pool if you're having a water birth, though.)

Reflexology

This alternative therapy involves massaging particular points of the feet and is said to work in a similar way to acupuncture, by tapping in to the body's energy channels and helping to release naturally occurring painkillers and reducing anxiety. Again, find a qualified practitioner to help you.

Hypnosis

Some people reckon you can think the pain of childbirth away – or at least distract yourself from it – through the art of hypnosis, or more specifically, 'hypnobirthing'. It's based on the theory that fear causes tension and tension makes pain worse, and involves putting the mind into a deep state of relaxation. To learn the techniques, you'll need to find a registered therapist – and put in lots of practice before the birth. There are also CDs available which claim to teach self-hypnosis.

Breathing techniques

Slow, rhythmic, deep breathing can help you relax during labour and you're more likely to cope with pain if you relax into it, rather than tense up. Breathing can also help you conserve your energy, and boost oxygen supplies to you and your baby.

- One recommended exercise is to focus on a two-syllable word, for instance, 'relax', and to repeat it in your mind in time to your breathing – 'reeeeee', as you breathe in, and 'laaax', as you breathe out. (You can use any word, but relax seems a good option.)

- You could also try counting while you breathe, or more simply, breathing in through your nose and out through your mouth.

- Trying to keep your shoulders loose and relaxed can help reduce tension, too.

- Your birth partner can get involved and help by breathing along with you.

As with other natural ways of coping with pain, you might find that deep breathing only takes you a certain distance.

Massage

Just like acupuncture and reflexology, massage is said to work by putting pressure on the body's energy channels and forcing out those endorphins. And massage just boosts relaxation and wellbeing generally – especially when applied with a bit of love and commitment from a willing birth partner. He (or she) could try gently rubbing your shoulders, to help reduce tension, or they could focus on the lower back, where the pain of contractions is often most intense. Ask him to use long, slow, rhythmic and fairly firm strokes or circles with his fingers, or the palm of his hands – you can let him know what feels good. He may also need to bear in mind, though, that some women find in labour that they can't bear being touched, and would rather be left to get on with their contractions alone. You might need to explain this in advance to him, to avoid any offence when you tell him you will punch his lights out if he doesn't take his effing hands off you immediately.

YOUR BIRTH PARTNER

Who's the person that will hold your hand and wipe your brow whilst you labour to bring your child into the world?

Usually, it will be your other half, if you have one. But not everyone wants to take their man into the labour room with them and not every man is keen to go. You may prefer to take a close female friend or relative with you, and in fact research shows this might not be such a bad idea, as you're more likely to have a natural birth with another woman in the room with you. Some women have two birth partners (that way, you can have one on each leg). You're unlikely to be allowed more than that in a maternity unit – although if you're having a home birth, there's nothing stopping you from making a party of it, should you want to. Another option available these days is hiring some professional help in the form of a 'doula' – these are trained birth assistants who offer practical and emotional support. If you're interested, find out more at Doula UK.

Whoever you choose, it's a good idea if your birth partner (often called a birth supporter these days) knows what to expect. It can be hard persuading a man to pick up a birth manual, but they need to know at least roughly what they're letting themselves in for, because if they don't, they may have a shock coming. (Although it's probably only in movies that male birth partners really do faint or require medical attention themselves, *Modern Girl* Jill does let on that her other half had to leave the delivery suite at one point, to get some 'fresh air'.) Equally, if you're booked in for a c-section (or even if you're not, but just as a precaution) he should also have a good idea of what this will involve.

He may decide early on that he's going to stay away from the 'business end' – and maybe you're keen for him to because you're scared it will put him off the sight of your nether regions for life. Of course, one or both of you may well change your minds about this. After all, it's a pretty amazing experience seeing your kid come into the world.

If in doubt, thrust this book at him and ask him to read the following list. It gives some ideas for useful roles a birth partner can play. (I've used 'he' throughout, for convenience.)

What your birth partner can do in advance of the birth

- Be sure he knows where the maternity unit phone number is – he might need to call them for you if you're bent double by contractions.

- Take responsibility for the journey to hospital by making sure the car's shipshape and full of petrol, and that he knows exactly how to get there (lots of people do a 'dummy run' beforehand, timing how long it takes on average. It's also a good idea to know about any roadworks that might stand in your way.) Checking out the geography and cost of parking at the hospital is a job with his name on it, too.

- Make sure your bag is put in the car (many a birth bag has been left behind in the commotion …)

- Have a clear idea of what your hopes are for labour and birth. You might not be in a fit state to be assertive about your desires when it comes to it. (A word of warning, though: make it clear that *you'll* be making all the ultimate decisions in the labour room. The last thing you want is a 'helpful' husband reminding you of your plans to avoid an epidural, when you've decided you really, *really* need one, after all.)

- If you're having your baby at home, it could be his job to order your birthing pool and, when it arrives, to be the person who assembles or inflates it.

THE PROFESSIONALS

We've all heard horror stories about midwives-from-hell. The ones who tell you off for not trying hard enough when you've been trying to push your baby out for an hour-and-a-half, or those that purse their lips and pretend not to hear you when you're screaming for an epidural. (And that's if you get a midwife attending you at all, what with all the understaffing issues that abound these days.)

The truth is: what you can expect from the midwifery and maternity services available to you when you give birth will vary hugely according to where you're having your baby. And of course, attitudes and abilities differ widely among individuals.

The majority of midwives and obstetricians are kind and able professionals who will want to help you have the best birth possible (I have absolutely nothing bad to say about any of the hospital staff who helped me during my births). But as with any service occupation, there will inevitably be some who disappoint (the difference is that, whilst it doesn't matter that much if your electrician or plumber turns out to be dodgy or deficient, it's a big deal if the person who's delivering your baby does).

It comes down to pot luck, really. Unless you're having a home birth, you won't have a choice about who attends you on the day itself. Nor is there much you can do about it if your labour happens to stretch across more than one shift and you're faced with a change of midwife halfway through. This can be off-putting – and downright annoying if you were getting on fine with whoever was helping you in the first place. Then again, it can go in your favour. 'I had two midwives during my baby's birth. The first was awful; our relationship probably not helped by the fact I kicked her when she did an internal exam,' says *Modern Girl* Sara of her experience. 'However the second was fantastic. She let me do my own thing and really helped me towards the end.'

One thing to be said, though, is that while the care you get during the birth of your baby will be influenced by what sort of midwife you get on the day, and how much pressure the unit is under, your own attitude (and your birth partner's) will make a difference – as *Modern Girl* Melanie found: 'I ended up arguing with the midwife because I wanted to have an epidural and she was trying to persuade me not to,' she recalls. 'She was one of those 'mother earth' types and was obviously not impressed that I wanted one. But I persisted, and finally got my wish.'

So, like Melanie, do be prepared to speak up, ask questions, and assert yourself if necessary.

Be prepared

Obviously, it's a good idea to be prepared by knowing as much as possible about having a baby. In particular (while you certainly shouldn't worry yourself unduly about them) there are all sorts of things that can occur during labour and birth that require special treatment, and it's a good idea to know in advance what they are so that, should anything happen during yours, you'll be well informed and confident about it. Chapter 9 of this book tells you all you need to know about the basics of birth – so make sure you look at it well in advance of your due date, rather than saving it as reading material for labour.

BIRTH BY PLANNED CAESAREAN SECTION

You may find out in advance of your due date that you're going to have a caesarean section (sometimes shortened to c-section). This could happen if your consultant has identified a medical need during your pregnancy and thinks it will be safer for you, your baby, or both of you, if you give birth through a surgical procedure rather than in the normal way. It'll be known as a 'planned' or 'elective' caesarean (rather than an emergency one – there's more about those on page 184). Whether planned or not, caesareans are relatively common: they account for around 20% of births in this country.

There's a number of reasons why an obstetrician may want to pencil in a c-section for a first-time birth:

- If you're suffering from pre-eclampsia (see page 48).

- If it's been found or is suspected that your baby's head is too big to pass through your pelvis.

- If your baby is in a breech (bottom first) or transverse (sideways) position and attempts to turn him round have failed (see page 210). (Although, it is possible to have a breech baby vaginally – see page 211.)

- If you're expecting twins or more, since there are more likely to be complications (although in some cases it is quite possible to give birth to twins in the natural way. Any more than two babies, though, and you'll be very strongly advised to go with the c-section). For more, see below.

- If you have placenta praevia (see page 17) – in other words, the placenta is partially or completely blocking the exit to the womb.

- If you have an infection – for instance genital herpes – that could be passed to the baby during a vaginal birth.

- If you have a chronic medical condition such as heart disease or diabetes which would make the strain of a normal labour potentially dangerous for you.

Some people think that too many c-sections are carried out these days by scalpel-happy doctors who are cutting up women without good reason. Generally, however, a consultant who's keen to book you in for a c-section will have the health and safety of you and your baby at heart. He or she must consult you and explain their reasoning, though, outline any risks and benefits, and certainly can't make any decision without your consent. If a c-section has been advised and you want to be certain there are no other options, you could always do a bit of your own research before signing the form.

You may also be subjected to hints from some quarters that if you miss out on a vaginal birth then you don't get to join that 'club'. Well, that's just stupid: if you're booked in for a c-section because your doctor thinks it's a good idea, it doesn't mean you've been in some way 'short-changed', or robbed of the chance to experience birth 'properly'.

" I agreed to a planned caesarean because my daughter was breech. But the way c-sections were covered in my antenatal class made me feel terrible about it: I felt a failure before I even had my baby! In fact, the surgeon found I have an unusual shaped uterus, and the cord was round her neck three times – I'd never have been able to deliver her vaginally, and without a caesarean, I wouldn't have my daughter. **"**
Jane

There are also certain advantages to an elective c-section: you know exactly when your baby will arrive so can plan accordingly; the birth itself will be less painful (although your recovery won't), and, unlike the average 'normal' delivery, you'll know exactly what's going to happen on the day.

Doctors won't automatically carry out a caesarean section without a good reason (at least, not unless you're 'too posh to push', and prepared to pay handsomely to avoid doing so). However, a small number of women – usually due to a fear of vaginal birth and its consequences – would rather their baby was born surgically.

Medical factfile: tokophobia

An extreme fear of giving birth, tokophobia was only recently identified as a medical condition (in 2000) and is thought to affect as many as one in seven women. If you suffer from tokophobia, counselling or some other treatment such as hypnotherapy may help you to overcome it. But if you are truly traumatised by the thought of a vaginal birth, then you should certainly relay your fears to your doctor: you should get whatever psychological support you need and, if your fears are genuine and serious, a birth by elective c-section if it's what you want.

❝ I had an elective c-section, and personally, I reckon it was the easy option. I loved it!❞
Katie

One thing's certain: physically speaking, a caesarean section is by no means the easy option. Statistically, they carry an increased risk of complications, including abdominal pain, bladder injury, excess bleeding, endometriosis (inflammation of the membrane lining of the uterus), a blood clot developing, a need for further surgery, readmission to hospital and various problems with future pregnancies (although plenty of women who have a caesarean go on to have subsequent babies naturally). There's also the potential for infection of the wound. Recovery times are longer, and you will have to stay in hospital for several days, or more, after the surgery. You may also be more at risk of suffering from birth trauma, a form of post-traumatic stress disorder that can, in a small number of women, kick in after childbirth. There's more on caesareans on page 184.

❝ A planned c-section wasn't the way I wanted things to go, but in the end I had no choice, so I had to make my peace with it. **❞**
Suvi

MULTIPLE BIRTHS

Some doctors will routinely recommend a planned caesarean section if you're having twins, because there's more risk of complications arising – policies and attitudes vary, depending on who's looking after you. However, it's quite possible for twins to be born in the normal way – and around half are.

Your chances of having twins vaginally depends on a number of factors. Their position is probably most relevant – if the 'first' twin is in a head down position, or both of them are, then you should be able to have a normal delivery (assuming there are no other problems, such as a low-lying placenta – see page 17). Of course, as with normal babies, twins can move around in the womb and change position, so this is a situation that you might be able to have reassessed closer to your due date. Occasionally, in a vaginal twin birth, the first baby is born in the normal way, but the second has to come out via a c-section, perhaps because he's in the wrong position or an emergency situation arises.

Twins are usually born slightly earlier than most, at around 37 weeks, because there's less room in the womb for them to move around, which means they're smaller on average than singleton babies and therefore a bit more vulnerable.

When twins are born, there'll usually be more people present in the delivery room – as well as an obstetrician and a midwife, there's likely to be one or two paediatricians (doctors who specialise in the care of babies and children), just in case.

PREMATURE BIRTH

If your baby is born before 37 weeks, his birth is considered premature – about one baby in every 10 makes their appearance before this point.

There are many reasons why your baby might be born early, either because you've gone into labour spontaneously or because your doctor has induced you or carried out a c-section because he feels it would be risky not to. Twins or more are likely to make an earlier than normal exit, since it becomes rather a squeeze when you're sharing a womb in the late stages; and a mum's age can be relevant, with older women of 35-plus slightly more at risk of premature birth.

Premature rupture of the membranes (in other words, your waters breaking early) is a common cause, and this can be triggered by a number of things, including infection or excess amniotic fluid. Often, there'll be warning signs that premature birth is a likelihood which a midwife or doctor will pick up on during your routine antenatal checks. One in three premature babies are delivered by c-section, because of an increased risk of complications.

Babies who are born before they're full-term can have health problems because they haven't had the chance to fully develop. They may have difficulty feeding, breathing, and regulating their own body temperature. They're also more prone to infection and other problems such as jaundice or anaemia.

The good news is that special care babies, even those born quite some weeks before they're due, have a good chance of survival these days because the care and equipment available in special care baby units is so advanced. Recent figures show that babies born as early as 23 weeks have a 20% chance of survival, while at 25 weeks they have a 67% chance of survival. By 32 weeks, almost all babies will survive without any major health problems.

If you go into labour early, you may be given an injection which can temporarily halt contractions, giving you time to get to the nearest unit with specialist facilities for premature babies, and for doctors to treat your unborn baby's lungs with steroids, which can help to mature them.

If you're bleeding, having contractions, your waters have broken or are leaking, or you are in any way concerned that you've gone into labour early, you should contact your midwife immediately, or – if you're really worried – call an ambulance or go straight to your maternity unit.

8

Ready for take-off:
preparing for your baby's birth

THE WAITING GAME

Once you leave the second trimester behind you, the novelty of pregnancy often wears off. You've ceased to wallow in the glow of people's congratulations, satisfied your cravings for Magnums, and find it hard to believe you face a further 12 weeks of growth. Round about now, most women start to find it's all become a bit of waiting game, with birth the ultimate goal at the end of it, and a host of new or worsening physical symptoms to fend off in the meantime. For some, it can reach proportions of downright misery. Fortunately, there's loads to take your mind off it all, as you busily prepare for your baby's arrival.

Check-ups in the last trimester

Prepare yourself for yet more clinic visits, as you'll have more antenatal checks in your final trimester – it varies according to area, but in theory you should be seen at 28, 31, 34, 36, 38 and 40 weeks. Your midwife should always measure your abdomen, to make sure your baby's growing at roughly the expected rate (if she's worried it's not, she may refer you for a scan, see page 17). And, from about 36 weeks, she'll probably have a good feel each time, to find out which way the baby is 'presenting', or lying. You'll also continue to have routine testing of your urine and blood pressure.

Labour lessons

If you've signed up for some (and you'll need to do so well in advance as they get booked up quickly – see page 22) your antenatal classes will usually begin somewhere between six and 12 weeks before your due date.

If you haven't bothered, or you didn't get a place on an antenatal course, don't fret: there's so much good information available for mums-to-be these days in books, magazines, or online and it's perfectly possible to do your own research.

One thing you won't get though is the opportunity to meet at least one person you'd consider having a coffee with once your baby's born (and, quite possibly, several). Most new mums (and it's not compulsory – some are happy to go it alone) find that knowing and being in touch with at least one other woman in the same situation is a vital aid to sanity in the weeks and months after birth (and a bit further down the line, it also gives you someone to escape to the pub with). So if you're not signed up to classes and you're worried about missing out on the social aspect, then you might want to try and make a few more in advance of the birth, perhaps by logging on to an online community.

HOW YOU'RE GOING TO FEED YOUR BABY

It's a good idea to ponder in advance how you plan to feed your baby. The vast majority of modern mums, according to the results of the Infant Feeding Survey of 2005, give breastfeeding a go (although rates do tend to drop pretty quickly from as early as a week in). If you don't know already, you'll no doubt soon be hearing lots about how breastfeeding represents the best nutritional start you can give a baby in life, for a variety of reasons. But it's important to remember it's not the only option. See the boxes on pages 194 and 196 for the pros and cons of both breastfeeding and bottlefeeding. At the end of the day, it's your decision and you shouldn't feel pressured either way.

As with your plans for birth, it's wise to keep an open mind.

Breastfeeding

Determination to do the 'right thing' for your baby, combined with pressure from certain quarters, can make successful breastfeeding seem like the holy grail of early motherhood. Unfortunately, many mums aren't prepared for the fact that breastfeeding can be bloody hard work to start with. Then when it doesn't work for them, they feel terrible. If you know you want to breastfeed it will help if you can look ahead with a positive attitude. But try to be realistic in your expectations – that way, you won't feel shattered if for some reason it doesn't happen. Turn to page 250 for more on the realities of breastfeeding.

Breastfeeding: pros and cons

Pros

- Breastfeeding is natural, therefore your milk will give your baby exactly the right nutrients, hormones and infection-busting antibodies that he needs.

- It's free.

- It's always on tap, with no sterilising, preparation, and heating of bottles to worry about.

- You don't have to go down to a cold kitchen to prepare night feeds.

- It may help to postpone the onset, or reduce the severity of, allergic conditions such as eczema.

- It's easily digested, making it less likely your baby will suffer from constipation or colic.

- It's said to enhance bonding. (It can make you feel very close.)

- It gives you a good excuse to sit down for long stretches.

- It's good for you – research shows it may help you reduce your chances of developing breast cancer and osteoporosis.

- It should help you lose weight, in theory, because the extra fat laid down in pregnancy is used to make breastmilk.

Cons

- The baby will probably need to spend more time feeding since breast milk is less filling.

- Only you can breastfeed the baby, so you can't delegate the job in the middle of the night or go out for a period of time since no one else can feed him.

- You may feel uncomfortable breastfeeding a baby in public.

- It can be difficult, frustrating, painful and stressful to get the hang of breastfeeding.

Preparing to breastfeed

You'll need to be practically prepared for breastfeeding. Have ready:

- Boxes of breast pads (leaking is just one of the joys – it's temporary, while your breasts adjust to your baby's demands, but you can get through dozens in the early weeks).

- Nipple cream. Sore nipples are par for the course, so have a tube of nipple cream on standby – midwives usually recommend Lansinoh, which is made from a pure form of lanolin.

- Breastfeeding bras. These can get very milky and smelly, so it's a good idea to have at least three or four.

- A selection of tops that either lift easily or unfasten down the front. Lots of high street shops now do these and you can't even tell they're designed for breastfeeding.

- Muslins are a real boon when breastfeeding as they mop up spills, and can be draped over your shoulder and your baby's dining area to provide a little privacy.

- A breast pump will be useful a bit later down the line if you want to express your milk into a bottle so someone else can feed your baby (however, don't try this for the first four to six weeks, to allow yourself a good chance to get breastfeeding established.)

There's not much you can do to prepare your nipples for the onslaught, and there's no point in either applying cream or putting yourself through the torture of 'nail brushing' them in a bid to toughen them up. Those babies will rise to the challenge when the time comes.

> 66 Looking back, I didn't do enough to prepare for breastfeeding. It was only after she was born that I read up on it. I wish I'd done more research earlier, but I was too focused on the birth. 99
>
> Rebecca

Bottlefeeding

The alternative to breastfeeding is of course bottlefeeding. Its main advantage is that it requires less of a commitment from you as your partner can share feeding duties. The reason there's not as much on bottlefeeding in this section isn't a purposeful bias – there's just less forethought needed.

Bottlefeeding: pros and cons

Pros

- It's easy to learn how to bottle feed.

- Anyone can bottle feed the baby.

- Father and baby get more chance to bond as he can take his turn bottle feeding.

- You don't have to worry about what you're eating (or drinking!) passing through to your baby.

Cons

- Formula doesn't have the same infection-fighting antibodies as breast milk.

- You have to get up in the night to sort out and warm the bottle.

- You need to spend time cleaning and sterilising, which can be a lot of work. If you travel, all this stuff has to go with you.

- Making up bottles can become a rather tedious chore.

- You have to pay for formula.

Preparing to bottlefeed

It's not difficult preparing bottles, although it's highly tedious, and the process can become somewhat soul-destroying when you make up your 16th that week. Cleanliness is everything so don't be tempted to cut corners and be prepared for a rigorous routine. Follow the manufacturers' instructions carefully, and make sure you get the quantities right. You will need:

- Some means of sterilising bottles, lids, teats, and formula scoops. A steam steriliser is the quickest and easiest method.

- Bottles, teats and lids.

- Formula: make sure you get the right age range – you want the one for newborns, not 'hungry baby' which could cause them to be seriously constipated, or 'follow-on-milk' (which most health visitors will tell you is an unnecessary bit of marketing, anyway).

SHOPPING NECESSITIES

At this stage, the answer is 'not much'. Parents-to-be are often superstitious about getting equipped for their baby too early, and the fact is that you don't actually need more than a few basics to start out with. Most people also find that they get lots of clothes (often beautiful, but somewhat impractical) as gifts. And you can always go shopping a bit later – online, if not in person.

On the other hand, you really do need to get your freshly discharged offspring something to wear, something to sleep on, and something to transport them in. And it makes sense to get the basics in with plenty of time to spare, just in case of a premature arrival. Besides, you're going to want to spend at least part of your maternity leave folding up sleep-suits, unfolding them, folding them, unfolding them, folding them, and so on …

Your baby's basic needs at the start are:

- Up to 10 vests and the same number of sleepsuits (get the sort with enclosed feet and you won't have to worry about keeping a pair of socks on him). Newborns really don't need any other sort of outfit: they want something comfortable, and you want something you can get on and off them easily (which you'll need to very frequently, since milky vomit and green poo stains abound).

- A cardigan for colder weather (perhaps two so you've always got one clean).

- A coat or jacket, unless it's a very warm time of year.

- A hat (ditto).

- Lots of teeny-tiny nappies. Disposables are the most convenient, but if the environment's a concern for you, and you can face the laundry issues, you could think about reusables. You'll also need a job lot of cotton wool; and some barrier or nappy cream.

- A cot or Moses basket. The basket is nice because it's cosier for a tiny baby and you can move it from room to room, which, since they sleep so much when they're tiny, is very useful. However, they only fit in them for three to five months, tops, and so they're not very economical. Most people borrow one – but for safety reasons, it's recommended that you always buy a new mattress. (There's more information on safe sleeping on page 270).

- Bedding. Get the fitted variety, and buy quite a few as they can get a lot of milky vom on them. You'll need one to two blankets depending on the time of year and these should be lightweight – the cellular sort, with holes in, are ideal. Some people swear by baby sleeping bags which, provided you're certain to get the right size, are suitable from birth.

- Muslins. The must-have accessory for new mums. Once the baby's born you'll probably be walking round with one permanently draped over your shoulder, to mop up the many and varied messes that your life is about to feature.

- A car seat. You won't be allowed to leave hospital (assuming you're going home in a car) without one of these. Buy new, or if you're taking on one that's second-hand, only accept from a good friend, in case it's been damaged in an accident, which could compromise its effectiveness.

- A pram and/or sling. The pram market's a huge one, and it's a pretty big purchase, so take your time and try before you buy. (I spent many a month bitterly regretting the monster three-in-one model we invested in without much thought – it required a degree in engineering to put it up or down, and was so heavy I could barely lift it into the car boot.) Features to look for are how light/sturdy it is; how well it 'handles'; how easily it can be collapsed and put up; and whether you've got enough room to store it at home. Slings are a popular transportation option for very young babies as they're less of a faff and less space-consuming than prams. They can also be useful if you need to get something done around the house, but your crabby baby refuses to be put down.

- Something to wash him in. You'll probably just 'top and tail' (see page 266) for a couple of weeks, anyway, and even then, a baby bath isn't really necessary as you can just use a large, clean washing up bowl until he's a little older and can be safely held in the big bath. However, a baby bath on a stand, or one that fits over the main bath, is a godsend if you have a bad back. Baby toiletries really aren't necessary for a newborn – in fact, their delicate skin could well do without it.

> " I wouldn't bother getting most of the baby stuff that's available. The amount you buy and never use is ridiculous. Plus, friends and relatives always want to buy you stuff so you can end up with five playmats and seven bouncy chairs – like toasters at weddings. I'd recommend buying as much as possible second-hand, or even just borrowing. "
> Claire

COPING STRATEGIES FOR THE FINAL STRAIT

You really don't need to paint the skirting boards. I say that because, in actual fact, I really *did* paint all the skirting boards in our house while on maternity leave with my first baby. And I'm still not sure why. So, with the benefit of hindsight, could I insist you resist the urge, if possible, to take on any major DIY or cleaning projects in the run-up to your baby's birth? Lots of women get a surge of energy in late pregnancy and feel compelled to remove dust from unseen corners and get a new coat of paint on the skirting boards as they await their baby's arrival, usually put down to the so-called 'nesting' instinct, but quite often because they're simply bored out of their minds during maternity leave.

Whether or not it's a real biological imperative, there's no doubt that it's tempting to try and get the house in order, because you won't have a chance once junior's your main priority. However, the real truth of it is that your baby won't actually give a toss what his immediate environment's like and, as you'll have more important stuff to worry about and really do need to conserve every ounce of energy you've got for the physical challenges ahead, you'd do well to take the same attitude.

For fairly obvious hygiene reasons, a clean(ish) kitchen is a good idea (especially if you're bottlefeeding), and it's useful to clear all floor surfaces of any tripping hazards. But really, major renovations and decorations during pregnancy are a waste of time: unless it's fulfilling a genuine need to entertain yourself, you'd be better off spending the last few months resting and savouring your remaining child-free moments. It's true you won't have much time to sort the house out after the birth, but then again, once your baby grows into a toddler, there'll be even less point, since he will wreck it in any case.

As for the nursery, make it look beautiful if it pleases you to do so. But otherwise, content yourself in the knowledge that your baby will probably be in with you for a while and, even once you've moved them into their own room, many years will pass before he or she takes any interest in interior design (if at all).

Things to do before your baby is born

- Have a good old tidy up, but don't obsess about the skirting boards and a designer nursery.

- Do a big shop of basics such as loo roll and staple foods, so you don't have to worry about shopping once you've brought your baby home. Make meals for the freezer, if you're that way inclined. But bear in mind that all the big supermarkets deliver – so if you don't get a chance or you can't be bothered to stock up, you're unlikely to starve.

- Get some sleep, a bit more sleep, and yet more sleep. You're not going to get a good night's kip for months (and possibly years) to come.

> 66 Get loads of sleep, as you never get it again; have lots of beauty treatments; read lots of magazines; make the most of drinking your tea and coffee hot – it always goes cold when you have kids. 99
> Coral

- Do some research into birth and think about how you hope yours might pan out (see page 167).

- Read up on babycare. Lots of new mums realise they were so busy reading about pregnancy and birth, they forgot to work out how to look after their baby. As they say – they don't come with instructions.

- Go out – for a meal, to the cinema: when your baby is born, your social life will die.

> 66 In the three weeks before the birth, I went to the cinema three times a week, always with coffee and muffins. It was so worth it – I've never been since. 99
> Sheridan

- Go for a 'babymoon' with your partner. Whether a proper holiday or a relaxing mini-break, it's a great idea to get away with your other half for a while – preferably with plenty of time to spare, so you don't have to worry about going into labour in a strange place (and bearing in mind that most airlines won't let you travel late in pregnancy). Some travel companies are actually marketing 'babymoons' now, and there's also a growing number of hotels and spas that offer what's described as a 'complete antenatal package'.

66 We'd planned to go out for a romantic meal on Valentine's Day, two weeks before my due date, but we couldn't get a table and had a candlelit meal at home, instead. I was somewhat relieved we weren't in a posh restaurant though as, when I stood up afterwards, my waters went with an almighty gush. 99
Claire

- Get your legs and bikini line waxed and your nails, face and/or hair done. OK, so it's not compulsory, but some women find it makes a huge difference to their state of mind. Book into a salon for professional help where necessary, though – you attempt to wax your own bikini line at your peril. They say it's a good idea to have your hair cut into an 'easy to maintain style', since you won't have time to go the hairdressers once your baby is born. Although slightly depressing, this is probably true.

66 I worried about being in labour with hairy legs. Everyone laughed at me and said that, when the time came, it would be far from my mind. Wrong! I can still recall lying there, legs spread, thinking, 'I'm so glad I shaved yesterday ... 99
Claire

- Practise some relaxation and breathing techniques, and some birthing positions. It's true this may make you feel slightly foolish, but it could help when the time comes and hey, it's passing the time isn't it? If you're hoping your birth partner will be on hand with a bit of pain relieving massage, get him (or her) to have a trial run – without the pain, it will probably be quite enjoyable

- Pack your hospital bag. It's a good idea to have this by the door ready to go at least a couple of weeks before your due date. (Try to put it somewhere you won't fall over it, though.)

Growing pains

Late pregnancy can be a time of much physical misery. You may well find some of your 'niggles' get even worse – and you may find that you get a whole new set.

- **Exhaustion.** Just lugging around all that extra weight is enough to make you tired. That's before you take into account the insomnia (see below). Don't do too much.

- **Discomfort.** Fully expect your entire posture to change towards the end of your pregnancy. If you've ever seen a woman clearly nearing the end point of gestation, tummy thrust out and legs splayed as she walks – or rather, waddles – you'll already have a good general idea of how your gait is likely to change. Your balance may also be shot, too.

- **Breathing difficulties.** As your womb expands, it puts pressure on the lungs, making it harder to breathe. There's not much you can do about it, but rest and take it easy whenever you get the chance.

- **Backache and pelvic pain.** This tends to increase in later stages as the added weight puts pressure on your spine and forces you into a curved posture. Try to rest, do some regular, gentle ab-strengthening exercises, stick to sensible shoes, and watch your posture.

- **Tummy pains.** As the ligaments stretch to support your growing uterus, it's normal to feel some pain and strain in your tummy area, although it can be a bit worrying if you're not sure what it is. Chat to your midwife – she'll almost certainly be able to put your mind at rest. You may also begin to experience Braxton Hicks (see page 214), or practice contractions, which feels like a tightening sensation across the tummy – in fact, these occur throughout pregnancy, but aren't usually obvious until the third trimester. Although generally passed off as 'painless', some women report that they're pretty uncomfortable towards the end.

- **Rib pain.** Caused by the womb pressing against the ribs, and also sometimes by your baby, bless his little football boots, attempting to bend it like Beckham inside you.

- **Leaky boobs.** Your breasts may leak a little colostrum – the golden, nutrient-rich pre-cursor to ordinary breast milk – during the third trimester. If it's bad, you'll just have to crack open the breast pads.

- **Indigestion and heartburn.** This can happen because your digestive organs are being thoroughly squashed by the lack of space. It may also affect your appetite. Try cold milk, or Gaviscon.

- **Insomnia.** An increasingly active baby and difficulty in trying to find a single remotely comfortable position means that getting a good night's sleep gets harder the nearer to your due date you get. There's only one way to get any comfort in bed in the late stages, and that's lying on your side, so inevitably you can start to yearn for a different position. And also of course, you'll have lots on your mind as you dwell on what lies ahead. (Round about now you might begin to start having some seriously weird dreams about birth, and your baby. It's normal.) Pillows will help – in particular, you'll find that one placed under your bump and one in between your knees can provide some relief.

- **Itchy tummy.** As your skin stretches over your growing bump, the result can be itchiness and irritation. A non-perfumed emollient like aqueous cream, or some calamine lotion, might help. But don't forget that extreme itching in the third trimester can be a symptom of obstetric cholestasis (see page 51), so keep an eye on it.

- **Swollen feet and hands.** Medically known as oedema, it's normal for water retention to worsen in this phase of pregnancy. However, it's linked to pre-eclampsia (see page 48), so it's a good idea to keep your midwife informed. Try to rest and put your legs up when you can.

66 I found the third trimester a miserable, soul-sapping, exhausting and tortuous experience: awful pelvic pain, horrendous insomnia, and the horrible sensation of your insides being kicked and your cervix being head-butted. Yuck. 99

Alison

Anyone for perineal massage?

Your perineum (in case you don't know) is the area between the vagina and anus, and during birth it inevitably comes in for a right old battering, very often tearing as the baby's head comes out. Some people reckon you can help to avoid this by using your fingers and a little oil to massage the area daily in the last three to four weeks of pregnancy – there's a specific technique, which your midwife can show you. If you do try it, make sure your hands are clean and your nails short, and choose a lubricant that won't irritate – wheatgerm oil is said to be the best (it's available from health food shops: if the assistant smirks, she knows what you want it for). One of the main problems of trying to massage your perineum is access: a huge bump can make this somewhat challenging. If so, you'll have to ask your partner to do it for you. (And this is where you find out just how much he loves you ...)

Raspberry leaf

Taking a regular dose of this herbal remedy in the last six to eight weeks before your baby's birth is reckoned to help stimulate the uterus and encourage a shorter labour. There's no scientific evidence to back this view, but some women swear by it. You can take it in one of two forms: either in a tablet or by infusing the dried leaves in hot water to make a tea – both are available from health food shops. Don't take raspberry leaf tea any earlier in pregnancy, though.

PACKING YOUR BAG

You'll need to get together a bag for your hospital stay and keep it by the door, at least a couple of weeks before your due date. Assuming things go without complication, you probably won't stay in hospital for longer than a day and night afterwards – lots of women feel very keen to get home and anyway, these days many hospitals are pressed for space.

However short your visit turns out to be, though, you're going to need a certain amount of stuff to see you through labour and birth, and for however long you hang around for afterwards. In fact, by the time you've got what you need together, you may find it fills three bags: one for labour, one for afterwards, and one for your baby. If you end up with so much labour luggage it's causing a blockage in your hallway, you might need to streamline it to just the essentials.

Stuff to pack for you

- **Something to give birth in.** Although most hospitals will provide a gown, you might feel more comfortable in something of your own. Make sure it's something you're happy to throw away again afterwards, which you will almost certainly want to once it's covered in blood, sweat, and afterbirth – an old, baggy t-shirt is ideal. Taking two is probably a sensible precaution, in case you need to change midway through.

- **Maternity towels.** These are not the same as ordinary sanitary towels, oh no – they're bigger, and more absorbent – so make sure you get the right ones for the job. You may also get through rather more than you imagined – so stock up with several boxes, and take at least one to hospital in case you have to stay a while.

- **Big pants.** You'll need some super-sized knickers to fit your big sanitary towels in. Buy a cheap multi-pack of new ones – you'll get good use out of them for a few weeks after the birth, after which you can chuck them. Take at least six pairs, as you'll probably be changing them frequently.

- **Nursing bra and breast pads.** Try to get measured for a bra as near to your due date as possible – but bear in mind you might also need one in a size up, as your boobs will get even bigger when your milk comes, two to three days after the birth (see page 259). For bottlefeeders, bottles and formula will usually be provided by the hospital (but check first. And obviously you'll need a good supply plus steriliser and bottles at home).

- **A front-opening nightie or two.** You'll want something nicer to slip into once you've taken off your blood and amniotic fluid-soaked t-shirt, and a front-opener's ideal for breastfeeding.

- **Comfy clothing to change into before leaving.** You'll still be very flabby, and every bit of you will ache. A loose, soft tracksuit should be just the job.

- **Toothbrush and toothpaste, and some basic toiletries.** There probably won't be anything in the hospital and one thing you're almost certain to want afterwards is a shower. So take shower gel or soap, and shampoo.

- **Hairbrush and make-up.** It may sound shallow, but some joker's bound to want to take pictures of you before you've left hospital and, chances are, you won't be looking your best.

- **Warm socks and/or slippers.** Hospital floors can be pretty cold. Some women also like to keep socks on during labour. (These can also end up covered in gunk, so, again, make sure it's a pair you're not attached to.)

- **Snacks and drinks.** Catering can be a hit and miss affair in maternity units, especially if you become hungry or thirsty in the middle of the night, so bring your own sustenance. You might feel hungry during labour – and you'll very likely be ravenous afterwards. Have something non-perishable in your suitcase, like crackers or cereal bars, and pop in fresh stuff like fruit just before you leave. Don't forget some cartons of juice or bottles of water, too.

- **Boredom busters.** Labour can be a long, drawn-out affair and frankly, it can get tedious. Take a good book, some magazines, or your iPod to help keep boredom at bay.

- **A camera.** This is one photo opportunity you won't want to miss.

- **Your mobile phone.** You'll want to text everyone you know with the news once the baby's born, and put in a call to any expectant rellies. Remember that hospitals generally have rules about turning mobiles off, though. You may also want to make sure you've got change for a payphone in case you can't get a signal.

- **Lip balm.** If you're planning on having gas and air, this is essential as you may get dry and cracked lips.

- **Sponge; water spray; stereo and your delivery music of choice.** All optional extras.

Stuff to pack for the baby

You won't need to take much to the hospital for your baby, other than several soft cotton sleepsuits and vests; a cardigan or jacket; a hat (depending on the weather); a blanket for the journey home; nappies and cotton wool.

Most important of all is the car seat: unless you're walking home, the hospital won't let you leave without one of these.

THE THINGS PEOPLE SAY

The bigger you become, and the closer to your due date you get, the more annoying the comments you can expect from other people. It's human nature to be fascinated by the sight of a woman's body as it carries out the awe-inspiring role it was designed for – and to be excited about the prospect of a new kid on the block. So try to be understanding when people want to give your belly a little stroke, or ask: 'Haven't you had that baby yet?' And hard though it may be, you must resist the urge to throw back a sarcastic reply like, 'Yes I have. The baby's at home and now I'm just really fat.'

If the touching bothers you, just ask them politely to refrain. As for stupid observations ('My goodness, you're that big and you still have four weeks to go?') and 'helpful' birth advice ('You'll be fine! I managed on gas and air alone'), try to take it with good grace. If you can't do that, just ignore them.

YOUR FEELINGS

Make no mistake, the final weeks of pregnancy can be a pretty miserable time emotionally, too. It's normal to feel utterly fed up with your condition and absolutely desperate to get your baby out. It's also quite usual to be terrified about what's ahead of you – and not just birth, which, let's face it is at least over within a day or two. Parenthood, on the other hand, is something you'll have to contend with indefinitely. Now *that's* scary.

> 66 I was fed up with feeling squashed internally by the twins, no room to breathe, sore legs, puffy everything – and remember, thinking it would be great if my face was the first thing people saw rather than the great big bump I was heaving around. 99
>
> Amanda

Aim to take your mind off your fears by filling your final baby-free weeks with stuff you won't be able to do soon and concentrating on all the positives – in a very short time, there'll be a third, rather adorable (if wearing) small person in the house. You might find a bit of relief from some gentle exercise helps you to relax. And you should try to spend some quality time with your other half, talking through any worries with him. He's probably scared, too, and could do with the reassurance himself.

Reading up on birth is important, because you need to be prepared, but equally you don't want to get too obsessed with what's ahead and become panic-stricken. Try thinking about something completely different, sometimes. See friends, or take in a good movie – whatever you did to enjoy yourself before the alien invasion (other than boozing).

66 I tried to enjoy the pregnancy and not wish that it was over. The best thing to do is relax and make the most of it while you have the chance. The baby will be with you soon enough. 99
Claire

YOUR BABY'S POSITION

From around 28 weeks, your midwife will start feeling your belly to check his position. By now, the majority of babies will have turned round to a cephalic, or head down position, ready for birth but some will be 'presenting' bottom or feet first (breech) and occasionally a baby will lie in a transverse position (sideways). Often, a breech or transverse baby will move round of his own accord in time for birth and, if not, he can sometimes be encouraged to wiggle round.

66 I felt impatient, huge, unsexy, uncomfortable. I spent most of the last few weeks on my birthing ball trying to turn the baby round and satisfying an intense satsuma craving. 99
Lara

You can also try and coax your baby round yourself. One trick is to lie on your back close to a wall, placing your feet high on the wall and then, using the wall for support, lifting your hips as high as you can (you can cushion your back, shoulders and hips with pillows). Try to spend 15 minutes doing this three times a day. You could also try spending as much time as possible on all fours, and wiggling your hips. Just don't try this in public.

It's not unusual for a baby who's turned to flip back again and if your baby remains steadfastly in the breech position by the time he drops down into the pelvis ready for birth (as an estimated 3% do), your consultant is very likely to advise a planned caesarean section. However, it could still be possible for a breech baby to born in the normal way if you're keen to give it a try, and there are no other complications. A persistent transverse position can signal other potential problems, though, such as a placenta praevia (see page 17), and so if you're baby's determinedly taking a sideways view of life by the very end stage of pregnancy, you'll inevitably have to undergo further investigation and prepare for the likelihood of a c-section.

Most babies with their head down will be in what's known as the anterior position as you approach your due date – in other words, with the back of his head facing your front. However, some end up the other way round, with the back of the head towards the spine. This can cause severe backache during late pregnancy and birth. It also means he'll be likely to take longer to drop into the pelvis, and then take his time trying to move round the right way before being born, causing an overdue and/or prolonged labour, with an increased likelihood of needing help with the delivery (see page 232). If you find out your baby's in a posterior position, you might be able to encourage him to swing round by keeping active and spending as much time as possible in upright standing or sitting positions, or on your hands and knees.

66 My son was breech for most of the third trimester, but he turned at 35 weeks when I was in the bath, leaving me feeling a bit sick. It was a bit like something out of Alien. 99

Sheridan

Engagement

At some point from around 37 weeks, and sometimes earlier for a first baby, your baby's head will 'engage'. In other words, the little monster drops down into your pelvis in readiness for birth. (This process is also sometimes known as 'lightening'). It can give your lungs and ribs relief, but may give your bladder and pelvis some grief instead. You can't win 'em all.

Your *absolutely* final checklist

OK, so are you ready for this? Don't forget to:

- Pack your bag, and your birth plan, if you have one.

- Have your maternity notes ready to take, if you've been keeping them at home.

- Make sure the house is reasonably shipshape and you've got a bit of food in the freezer.

- Keep the car in working order and full of fuel (this one's for him).

- Put your birth partner/person responsible for transporting you to hospital on red alert (hint: they'll need to stay sober so they can drive at short notice, and they need to always be at the other end of their mobile).

- Have numbers for your midwife/maternity unit in a prominent place.

- Have a car seat and the few basics your baby will need ready.

- De-fuzz your legs and bikini line. A girl's got to have some dignity, after all.

9

Labour day(s): what happens when you give birth

So here we are. You thought the piles and the backpain were bad, well, this is the bit that really hurts (usually). It may be easier said than done, but please try not to brick yourself at the thought of labour. Yes it hurts, yes it can go on for a bloody long time, and yes it can often turn out to be a bit more complicated than you might hope for. But with a tiny, tiny minority of exceptions, births in this country almost always work out all right in the end.

You can't know what having a baby's like until you've actually had yours. But you can get a rough idea of what's coming and prepare yourself to some degree simply by having a good old read of the following chapter. I've tried to be as honest as possible. And I've gone with the stance that it's better to know what will or could happen than to be unprepared and then wonder WTFs going on when the time comes.

YOU'RE NEARLY THERE …

Your body may start to gear itself up for labour for a few days or even weeks before it actually kicks off. So although they can be useful indicators that the time's approaching, there'll usually be no need to panic at the onset of any of the following signs. Give the maternity unit a quick call if you're worried – the duty midwife will probably tell you to make a cup of tea, put your feet up, and wait for your baby in as relaxed a way as possible.

What to look out for

- An increase in or thickening of vaginal discharge. It's normal to have some throughout pregnancy, but towards the end it can increase, caused by the baby's head pressing on the cervix.

- Backache, or a period-pain like feeling.

- A 'show'. This is when the jelly-like plug (it looks like heavy discharge and will often be streaked with blood, which can be a little alarming) that seals the cervix comes away. It can do this some days or even a couple of weeks in advance of labour beginning, or it may not happen until the last minute.

- Stronger Braxton Hicks. These 'practice' contractions actually occur for a long time before your due date – it's just that they don't always become noticeable until later and can become really quite intense, and uncomfortable even, in the final few weeks. Lots of first-timers wonder if the Braxton Hicks they're experiencing are real contractions. (If you're not sure they're strong enough to be real, the truth is that they probably aren't.)

- A bout of diarrhoea. This can happen sometimes in the 24 hours before things kick off, as Mother Nature clears out the bowels in readiness for labour.

GOING PAST YOUR DUE DATE

It's not particularly unusual for an EDD to come and go without so much of a hint of your waters breaking or contractions starting. Normal pregnancies can continue for up to 43 weeks – and due dates are very often inaccurate, anyway.

Going past your due date can be an anticlimax, and a considerable strain when you feel your tummy's already at bursting point. Both my babies hung on in there for two weeks beyond their expected birth-day, so I know the suspense can be crippling. Although frustrating, it's nothing to be alarmed about. However, your maternity team will be keeping a careful eye on you from then on because in pregnancies that go beyond 41 weeks, the risk of a baby being stillborn or becoming distressed starts to rise slightly.

If there's no sign of your baby by your due date, you'll usually be offered a 'membrane sweep' before anything else is suggested – your midwife or doctor will run a finger round the inner edge of your cervix to encourage it to start dilating. It can be uncomfortable, may make you bleed a bit, and can also cause cramps, so if you're booked in for one, don't have anything else planned for the rest of the day.

If this doesn't work, you'll usually be offered a day in the next week to have your labour induced – in other words, to get things going by artificial means. Most doctors will be keen for this to happen within 14 days of your due date – even if your pregnancy has been normal and there are no other risk factors. They should explain why they want to induce and what the risks and benefits could be. But you should still be offered the chance to wait for labour to start naturally if you prefer. If you do choose to wait, your doctor will probably want to see you frequently – possibly daily – to check that your baby's doing OK.

It's very normal to hope to avoid induction. For one thing, it will mean kissing goodbye to any plans you had for a natural birth, and for another, it could mean a very abrupt and intense start to labour pains (for which you

may need to consider some heavy duty pain relief, such as an epidural).
You don't have to have an induction if you don't want one (your labour
will start at some point – it has to!) but your doctor will recommend it
if he's concerned about you or your baby. Although the most common
reasons for induction is a simple matter of being overdue, other possible
reasons for it include:

- There are signs that your placenta has stopped working efficiently, or
  it is coming away, which could affect the oxygen supply to your baby.

Natural ways to encourage labour

Rumour has it you *might* be able to put a rocket under your baby's
arrival with the following methods. The only evidence that any of them
work is anecdotal rather than scientific. Still, you've nothing to lose
(and in some cases, a fair bit of fun to be had) in trying. Steer clear of
these altogether if you've had any complications.

- **A hot curry.** If eating spicy food really does work as a way to bring
  on labour, then it's probably something to do with a laxative effect
  that stimulates the uterus as well as the bowel. There's no scientific
  evidence whatsoever that it works, but still, as you might not get to
  go out for a curry for a while once your baby's born, you may as
  well get one in while you can. Don't attempt to have a really hot
  one if you're not used to it – this isn't the time for a stomach upset.

- **Hot sex.** It's unlikely a good hard shag in itself will bring on labour,
  although the theory is based in scientific evidence, since sperm
  contain prostaglandins which are said to soften the cervix, and the
  hormone oxytocin – which stimulates contractions – is released
  when a woman comes. You shouldn't have sex once your waters
  have broken, because of the risk of infection.

- **Nipple tweaking.** Stimulation of the boobs aids the release of
  oxytocin, same as when you orgasm. The idea is to use your palm
  and rub both nipple and areola (the dark skin surrounding the
  nipple) in a circular motion. You need to be pretty committed, since

---

- Your waters have broken and there's an increased risk of infection.

- Your baby's growth has slowed or stopped.

- You have an existing medical condition such as diabetes or heart disease, or a pregnancy condition such as pre-eclampsia or gestational diabetes and your doctor thinks your baby (or you) would be safer out than in.

There's more about induction on page 224.

---

it's reckoned that you need to do this for an hour three times a day if it's actually going to work. (That's a lot of tweaking.)

- **Pineapple.** This tropical fruit contains the enzyme bromelain which is said to boost production of prostaglandins. You'd have to eat it in large quantities to get enough of the stuff to be effective, and by then you're probably looking at the same sort of effect as a hot curry.

- **Raspberry leaf tea.** Although this might be helpful in preparing the uterus for birth if taken in the last month or two (but no earlier) of pregnancy, it's a myth that a single dose or cup will trigger labour. (It was pure coincidence, I'm sure, that my waters went pop an hour after I supped on a cup of the stuff ...)

- **Castor oil.** An old wives' favourite, and another method based on bowel stimulation, but not really to be recommended as castor oil tastes foul and could leave you nauseous, dehydrated, and suffering from diarrhoea and painful bowel cramps.

- **Reflexology, aromatherapy, homeopathy and acupuncture.** Practitioners of all these alternative therapies claim they might give a natural kickstart to labour. There's no science to back those claims, but they might be worth a try if you've got an open mind. Contact a qualified practitioner first – and be prepared to pay.

- **Long walks.** Moving around and keeping upright could help for the simple reason that gravity might jiggle your baby further down towards your cervix. Take a stroll if you're up to it, but don't try anything too strenuous at this point – you need to save your energy.

WHAT HAPPENS WHEN YOUR WATERS BREAK

At some point, the sac of amniotic fluid surrounding your baby will burst and spurt or dribble out from your vagina – this is commonly known as your waters breaking. For most women, this doesn't happen until after contractions have begun and labour has started (and sometimes they're popped for you by a doctor or midwife as part of an induction process).

However, for about one in 20 women, waters break before labour starts. So if your waters go but your contractions haven't yet begun, it's a sure sign that they soon will. You should give your midwife a call if it happens to you. You'll probably be asked to go in for an assessment because, once your waters go, there's an increased risk of an infection travelling up your vagina and reaching your baby.

You may be offered an induction at this point, or given the option to take a 'wait and see' approach, in which case you'll be sent home but asked to be vigilant for possible signs of an infection, such as a high temperature or changes to the colour and smell of your amniotic fluid. In nine out of 10 cases, labour starts within 24 hours of waters breaking early. If it goes beyond that, an induction will probably be recommended as the infection risk will continue to increase.

It's a bit of cliché, but it's true that your waters can break without any warning, which might cause a slight embarrassment if you're in public. 'Mine went while sitting on a friend's mum's white sofa,' confesses *Modern Girl* Katie. 'Thankfully she was lovely about it.'

Although the experience can sometimes feel like a huge, watery gush, it's not as much as you imagine – and some women find it amounts to no more than trickle. The fluid should be very pale in colour or clear, sometimes with a little blood, or a pinky tinge. If there's any green or brown in it, or it is very bloody, call the maternity unit straight away to let them know. They'll probably want you to go in for an assessment, as this could signal a potential problem.

" When my waters broke, it was the weirdest feeling. I thought for a moment I'd wet myself! I was shocked at how much comes out, and for how long. "
Melanie

HOW MUCH DOES IT HURT?

The start of proper contractions means the first stage of labour is definitely underway. Contractions – also known as labour pains – are what happen when the muscles of the uterus flex as it works to open up the cervix (the neck of the womb), from where your baby will soon be making his exit. They're almost always mild to start with (you may even mistake them for Braxton Hicks) and spaced far apart – perhaps every 20 minutes. This stage, known as the latent phase, can go on for ages – a whole day or even two is not unusual, particularly in a first birth.

Overall, it's hard to say how long a first-time labour's likely to be, as it varies so much, but between 12 and 24 hours is usually cited as average (with many of the *Modern Girls* reporting labours longer still than that).

It's a good idea to stay upright and active if it happens during the day, and to try and sleep or doze if it's night-time. Try to have something to eat and drink, too, if you can, to boost your strength – although admittedly some women do feel off their food around now (and even sometimes feel sick or vomit during this phase). This is also a good time to have a bath, to help you relax and which may also soothe the pain of the contractions. Other ways to pass the time in as relaxing a way as possible include going for a gentle walk, or watching something you love on telly, listening to your favourite music, and getting your other half to give you a massage. A good tip for coping with the milder pain of early labour is to pop a couple of paracetamol, which should take the edge off a bit.

What do contractions feel like?

It's really hard to describe what contractions feel like, as they can vary so much from one woman to another. Some liken them to intense period cramps; others say they are far, far more painful than that. Some women feel them in their abdomen, others in their back. And some women find they are really quite bearable, even without any pain relief, while others are shocked at just how agonising they are.

Descriptions from the *Modern Girls* vary:

- 'A fucking band of steel-tightening pain.' (Rebecca)

- 'Like someone punching you in the tummy.' (Louise)

- 'Like having your internal organs drilled into.' (Alison)

- 'Huge pressure, like I needed to do the biggest poo in the world.' (Judy)

- 'Like someone thinking your insides were an orange they are trying to squeeze.' (Nina)

- 'Like hot knives slicing through you.' (Isla)

- 'At each stage, I thought the pain could not get any worse. Boy, was I wrong!' (Jenny)

And if all that sounds scary, take comfort in the thoughts of these *Modern Girls*:

- 'An intense tickle.' (Melanie)

- 'No worse than normal period pain.' (Claire)

- 'Boringly monotonous.' (Kelly)

- 'Like back pain – I felt nothing across the front.' (Zoe)

- 'Painful but over very quickly.' (Louise)

- 'It didn't hurt as much as I thought it was going to!' (Mel)

So there you go – I told you it was variable. One thing most women do agree on, though, is that if you relax rather than tense up through contractions, you'll be able to cope with them better.

Things that could be a worry in early labour

There's no need to go in to hospital or even call the maternity unit during early labour if your contractions are well spaced and you're coping OK. However, you should call your midwife straight away if:

- You're bleeding heavily (although a certain amount of blood as part of your 'show' is normal).

- Your waters have broken and are stained with a green/brown substance – this is likely to be meconium (your baby's poo) and could indicate that he's in distress, or be a sign of an infection.

- You have pain in your tummy that's constant (as opposed to coming and going, which is what contractions do).

- You have sudden or severe headache or vision disturbances (it could be a sign of dangerously high blood pressure).

- You don't think your baby is moving any more, or your baby seems to moving around in a frenzy.

WHAT IF MY BABY WON'T WAIT?

As most first-time labours last at least a day or two, you should have loads of time to work out if you're actually about to have your baby before heading to the maternity unit (and still have oodles more time to spare when you get there). Once in a while, though, a first-time mum can be taken by surprise with a very short labour and a baby who arrives before she's even had time to pick up the telephone. If it happens to you, here's what to do:

- Try to call someone who can be with you quickly, if you don't have anyone there already.

- Ring the emergency number on your notes. They'll make sure someone comes to you. If you can't find the number, dial 999 and ask for an ambulance. Make sure the front door's open so they can all get in.

- Try to find some towels – one to save your carpet, and a large clean one to wrap your baby in.

- Kneel with your head on your forearms and keep your bottom as high up in the air as possible. Resist pushing if you can. Try breathing in a pattern of three short pants and a long blow. This can help delay things a bit.

- If you can't resist the urge to push and your baby starts to make its way out before anyone's got to you, don't panic. Hold on to him, and carefully check to make sure the cord isn't looped round his neck (ease it gently back over if it is, but don't pull it).

- Once your baby's all the way out, wrap him up to keep him warm. There might be mucus or fluids in his nose preventing him from breathing properly, which you can push out by stroking down the sides of his nose.

- Place the baby on his front across your belly with his head lower than his body to allow any remaining fluid to drain out, and firmly rub his back with the towel.

- Don't attempt to cut the cord – the professional who comes to your aid will sort that for you, but do cuddle him close and try putting him to your breast. Your placenta should follow soon afterwards, still attached to the cord.

'ESTABLISHED' LABOUR

Eventually the contractions will begin to come more often, be longer-lasting, and feel more intense. Once they're coming thick and fast, every four to five minutes, say, you're considered to be in 'established' labour.

Even now, you're very likely to be between six and 12 hours away from having your baby. Generally, midwives encourage you to stay at home for as long as you can before coming in to hospital, assuming there are no problems, and that you're coping OK with the pain. After all, if you've got to hang around waiting, you may as well do so in the comfort of your own home.

Make a call to the unit once your contractions are coming regularly, every five to six minutes or so. You could then be advised by the duty midwife to come in (especially if your waters have broken by then), or you may be advised to stay put a while. If you do go in, and the midwife establishes that you've still got a long way to go, you might be sent home again.

IN HOSPITAL

If you've been advised to go in, or you turn up anyway, a midwife will take your pulse, temperature and blood pressure and check your urine. She'll feel your abdomen to check the baby's position, and listen to the baby's heartbeat. Then she'll probably carry out an internal examination on you to see how things are going: as labour progresses, the cervix gradually dilates (opens up), and when the midwife examines you she's checking to see how far along this process has got. If she says you're '1cm dilated' then you're only just at the start. Labour isn't considered to be established until the cervix is 3cm–4cm dilated, and you're not 'fully dilated' and ready to go until it opens up to 10cm.

Until you're coming close to the moment of pushing your baby, your midwife will probably leave you and your birth partner to pass the time together in the delivery room. She'll pop in from time to time to check you're OK, to listen to the baby's heart rate, and to see if you're any closer to being fully dilated. Meanwhile, move around if you can and put your breathing and massage techniques to use to help you cope with the pain of contractions. But pipe up if, at any point, you're not coping with the pain and you need something to help you. There should be a button you can press to alert your midwife.

Electronic monitoring

Usually the midwife will keep a close check on your baby's heartbeat during labour with a hand-held monitor. But in some cases – if your pregnancy or labour is considered high risk for some reason, or a complication has arisen – she may want to wire you up to a piece of equipment called an electronic foetal heart rate monitor. This works by using two sensors attached to a machine that strap on to your belly with elastic belts, and can read your baby's heartbeat, and contractions. From this, your midwife or doctor can get a printout of this information in the form of a graph, and they can use it to see how your baby's coping during your labour.

Although reassuring and painless, the drawbacks to electronic monitoring are that it makes moving around and changing position difficult and it can make you feel like the subject of a science experiment. You might be more comfortable sitting in a chair while you're being monitored, rather than lying on a bed.

BEING INDUCED

About one in five women in this country end up having their labours artificially induced. If an induction is suggested, you should be given a full explanation as to why, and the risks, benefits, and alternatives, and given time to think about and discuss it before making a decision. You should then be told about the different ways in which your labour might be given a helping hand.

There's no set way for an induction to proceed – it could make things happen very quickly; you could end up waiting for many hours (and even a couple of days) for action; and in some cases, it may not work at all (after which, the usual route will be caesarean section – this can be pretty demoralising news if you've already spent an exhausting couple of days on the induction trail.)

What does induction involve?

The first attempt at inducing labour will usually involve you having prostaglandin. This is a synthetic version of the very same hormone that's released naturally in labour (and yes, from semen) to soften the cervix. They can be given in the form of a tablet, pessary or gel that's inserted into the vagina. One dose may not work, and sometimes a second or even third dose will have to be given. And it's quite possible they won't work at all. If they do, you've had a result, because it's a gentler method than what comes next and, in theory, your contractions shouldn't be any stronger than they would in normal labour.

If nothing happens (usual in about half of cases) your midwife or doctor may attempt to speed things up further by breaking your waters. This is done by inserting a small hook-like instrument into the vagina and making a small tear in the membranes – it's not supposed to hurt but may cause you some discomfort.

If this doesn't work, you'll be offered the next stage – Syntocinon (which is the artificial form of oxytocin, the natural hormone that triggers contractions), given via a drip into a vein in your hand or arm. So, all in all, your ability to move around will be very restricted. A drip has other major disadvantages, too – it can cause rapid and very strong contractions (so you may well need an epidural to cope with it) and it can put your baby under stress, so your baby will need continuous electronic monitoring.

66 I went in for the induction at 9am Monday morning, 3cm dilated. I was monitored for three hours but progress was slow and I was already utterly knackered. I managed to utter the immortal words 'can't you just break my waters?,' and within seconds of the midwife doing so, the contractions I'd been just about dealing with went from ouch to OOOUUUUUCH and I found myself in floods of tears, begging for an epidural. 99
Lara

HOW YOU MIGHT ACT IN LABOUR

Research has shown that keeping active and upright can make labour easier. So walking around (some women find they cover miles), bouncing on a birthing ball, getting down on all fours and wiggling your hips from side to side, or draping yourself in different ways over chairs, beanbags, or mats, could all help you find a bit of comfort and relief from the pain. You won't need to feel self-conscious about doing any of these things, even if you do suspect you look like a mad woman in the process: the staff will have seen it all before.

The position that you actually give birth in is said to make a big difference, too. Lots of women find crouching on all fours, or kneeling, squatting, or standing with support from a birth partner, are more comfortable and natural stances. And it makes sense when you think about it, because you'll be getting a helping hand from gravity.

If you feel strongly that you'd like to be free to move around or to experiment with different positions, it's something you could write in your birth plan. Be prepared to take the initiative in finding out what's comfortable for you when the time comes – how much encouragement you get to take control of your own position could depend on where you're giving birth, and who's assisting you. But bear in mind it's your body – you can put it anywhere or anyhow you choose.

EFFING AND BLINDING

There's a time and a place for everything, and the delivery room is not the place, nor delivery the time, for social niceties. Fact is, you may find yourself acting in a less-than-sedate way during labour. Different women respond in different ways but the truth is, it's such an extraordinary experience that you'll more than likely surprise yourself with some fairly extraordinary behaviour. 'I never, ever swear normally, but with every contraction, I was shouting 'fuuuuuuuuuck' at the top of my voice,' says Sarah. 'I was at home for quite a lot of my labour – so I did offer apologies to the neighbours afterwards!'

It's very common to let rip whatever extremes of emotions you're feeling on whoever's in the room with you – and you should perhaps point this out to your birth partner *before* the big day, so he's psyched up for the possibility of being insulted. (Midwives won't usually take it personally if you're rude to them – they're pretty well used to it.) 'There was a point in labour where I told my husband to fucking go away,' admits *Modern Girl* Jayne. Lucy recalls, 'My other half was a brilliant birth partner, but when I turned round in the midst of a painful contraction only to catch him taking a bite out of a chicken tikka sandwich whilst staring into space, I flipped – and called him something very rude indeed.'

❝ I found the contractions so overwhelming I wanted everyone and everything else to go away, including my poor husband. He was all set to encourage me, hold my hand, massage me, all that stuff and I just told him to leave me alone!**❞**
Sara

Finally, bear in mind that you may feel a need to transfer your pain, which is potentially bad news for the poor sod who's offered to be your punchbag (err, sorry, I mean birth partner). Beware of digging your nails in so hard it draws blood …

Whatever surprising things you do in the throes of labour, you don't have to feel embarrassed about it. (And you know, you probably won't. In fact, you probably won't give a flying *fuuuuuuuuuuuck!*)

❝ To be completely honest, the only thing that helped me to get through it all was to get naked, scream the room down, bite my lips to pieces, and grab at my boobs with every contraction. I didn't expect myself to act how I did, but my body just took over.**❞**
Louise

What your birth partner can do for you during labour and delivery

- Keep you entertained (or just provide company) if you're enduring a long, boring wait for action.

- Massage your back to help ease the pain.

- Fetch you snacks, drinks, or anything else you need.

- Help keep you cool by sponging or spraying your face.

- Offer words of encouragement and support.

- Speak up or ask questions if something's happening you're not keen on or sure about (but only if you give them the nod first …).

- Provide support if you want to give birth kneeling, squatting or standing up.

- Let you know all's going well from his vantage point down 'the business end'.

- Keep a low profile and his mouth shut if you need him to!

" My husband was really involved throughout, and incredibly supportive. When I was in pain he knew what I wanted and communicated with the midwives for me. He drew the line at examining the placenta, though. I can't think why. **"**
Jane

HERE COMES YOUR BABY

In between the first and second stages of labour there sometimes comes a brief phase known as 'transition'. Contractions are incredibly intense and coming thick and fast, and you may feel shaky or sick, confused, distressed, and at the end of your endurance. It means you're close to the end though, and you're about to enter the second stage of labour: pushing out your baby.

As your baby's head moves right down through the cervix towards the vagina, you might feel a very intense pressure in your bum – almost as though you need an almighty poo. And you'll probably experience an overwhelming urge to push (you might hear this referred to as 'bearing down'), but if it's not yet time to do so, because the cervix isn't fully dilated, your midwife will ask you to hold back. You can help counter the urge to push by breathing in short puffs or pants.

Pushing

When the time's right, your midwife will want you to push with each contraction, and she'll guide you in doing this. A lot of mums report that they weren't quite sure how to do the pushing, and the piece of advice on this that crops up most often is to 'push like you're doing a poo', that is, through your bottom rather than through your fanny. Once the head begins to appear, you may want to put your hand down to feel it, or even take a look with the help of a mirror. Your midwife will urge you to stop or slow your pushing, breathing out in puffs, if it helps, so she can guide the baby out slowly, which will minimise the risk of your perineum tearing. Once the baby's head is out the hard work is done: you should only need to give another push to get the body out.

In some births, a baby will pop out relatively quickly and easily, but in others it's a truly knackering process that can take some time – up to an hour, sometimes longer still. If you're not comfortable at any point, get the help you need to change position.

Sometimes, in spite of your best efforts, your baby won't budge – perhaps because he's got himself into an awkward position, his head's too big to get through the birth canal, or your contractions have ceased to be strong and effective. When this happens, your doctor might suggest that using forceps or vacuum extraction (ventouse) to help him out (see below).

How much is this going to hurt my vagina?

Unless you're still benefiting from the effects of an epidural, you'll find that pushing your baby out stings pretty considerably – hardly surprising, really, when you weigh up the size of your baby's head against the size of your vagina. However, if you've already been through a long labour and many hours of agonising contractions, the truth is you'll probably find this the easy bit.

Lots of women suffer a torn perineum whilst pushing their baby out. Although this sounds horrendous, the reassuring truth is that at this stage of birth you're usually so focused on (and amazed by) your baby's entry into the world, you don't really notice the pain. If the tear is a small one, it will probably be left to heal on its own. If it's deep, though, it will have to be sewn up. For more on that, see the section on episiotomy, below.

Could I poo myself when I'm pushing?

This is one of those things that can cause a certain amount of advance horror among first-timers. It's only later that you will realise the truth: if you poo yourself during labour – which you might, because of all the pushing – it will be the *absolute least of your worries*. Farts and urine may also make their escape. Fear not, in any case: your midwife will be on the alert and will wipe any mess away, pronto, so you might not even notice. (And if you happen to poop yourself whilst in the birthing pool, you'll get to find out what that little fishing net's for …).

YOUR BABY'S OUT!

Once your baby's born, the midwife will quickly look him over and make a speedy routine assessment of his breathing, skin colour, heart rate, muscle tone and reflex response, known as an Apgar score or test. Occasionally, a baby will need his passages suctioned and sometimes a little extra oxygen, in order help him breathe.

The midwife will probably then pause to wipe some of the slimy mix of blood, amniotic fluid, and vernix your baby's likely to be covered in, before handing him over for a cuddle – this 'skin-to-skin' contact is seen as a good way of calming your baby, promoting bonding, and helping to get things off to a good start if you're going to breastfeed. Meanwhile, the umbilical cord will be clamped and cut and this is one small way in which your partner can play an active part in your baby's arrival – although if he's squeamish, he might prefer to forgo this option. You'll also get stitches now, if you need them. You may feel high as a kite at this point, or you may feel drained and slightly depressed. Both are normal.

Don't be surprised if your baby looks kind of hideous. As well as being rather slimy, newborns can be hairy, blotchy, somewhat swollen, squinty-eyed, and pointy-headed. Luckily, he'll be beautiful to you.

Delivery of the placenta

It's not quite over. While you're focusing on your new baby, contractions (though thankfully milder ones) will continue as your body prepares to expel the placenta, usually described as the size of a small dinner plate, often with a little more pushing needed from you. This is the third stage of labour.

This process should happen naturally within an hour or so of birth (and if you're keen for a natural delivery of the placenta, it's something you could put in your birth plan). However, it's common these days to be given an injection to speed things up and reduce the chances of excessive bleeding, known as postpartum haemorrhage (PPH), occurring. This is known as a 'managed' rather than a natural third stage and involves the midwife placing a hand on your belly and gently pulling the cord with the other to remove the placenta, usually within about five minutes of birth. (It may well cause you a bit more discomfort, but it won't be anything like as painful as pushing out your baby.) If you decide to let the placenta come out of its own accord and this process is prolonged, or it causes you to bleed heavily (which it might), your midwife might again suggest an injection to move things along.

Sometimes (in about 2% of births) all or part of the placenta is left behind because it's still stuck to the wall of the uterus – known as a retained placenta – and if it's not removed, it could also lead to a haemorrhage. If this happens the midwife will probably try to give it a tug to try and ease it out, but if it's still not coming you might need a small surgical procedure, known as manual removal of the placenta. For this, you'll need a local anaesthetic such as an epidural (or a top-up, if you had one for the birth, anyway), and you'll be taken to an operating theatre.

You may or may not be interested to sneak a look at your placenta – it's played a pretty important role over the last nine months, after all. Or perhaps you'll want to take it home and carry out a symbolic burial of it under a tree in your garden; something mothers in Malaysia do.

Since it's said to taste a bit like liver and contain properties that help ward off postnatal depression, you may even want to borrow a controversial recipe from telly chef Hugh Fearnley-Whittingstall and make placenta pâté from it. (Add shallots and garlic, flambée, puree, and serve on foccacia bread.) My advice would be to let your midwife dispose of it. And if you do dish up placenta as a side order, don't invite your mates.

AN ASSISTED DELIVERY

If your baby needs help to be born because he's stuck, or if you're getting too exhausted to eject him on your own steam, you may end up having an assisted birth. This means the obstetrician will use either forceps or a vacuum extractor (ventouse) to get a good hold of your baby and ease him out. Forceps are curved tongs that look a bit like a large pair of salad servers. If these are used, you'll need to have an episiotomy (see below), to allow room for the forceps to fit up you and round your baby's head. A ventouse or vacuum extractor is more like a sink plunger: it has a plastic or metal cap which fixes to your baby's head, and a vacuum pump which is used to cause a suction effect. While both of these things look and sound terrifying, it might help to bear in mind that they're pretty commonly used and, unless he's fresh out of medical school, your obstetrician will be experienced in wielding them.

Vacuum extraction is more common and is the gentler option of the two as it doesn't usually require an episiotomy and you're less likely to suffer any damage or pain as a consequence, but forceps are more likely if your baby is facing the wrong way and needs turning. Babies born with assistance will usually bear temporary marks as a souvenir: forceps can leave red marks on the temples, while vacuum extraction can cause swelling and a misshapen head – this goes down within a few days, and will have sorted itself out completely within a week or two.

In either case, you'll need to lie on your back and have your feet placed in stirrups. You'll also need pain relief in the form of a local anaesthetic or epidural. Usually, a doctor will try one of these methods, but not both. If it doesn't work, he'll then suggest a caesarean section.

There's a school of thought that intervention techniques like these are too often carried out unnecessarily, robbing women of their chance to deliver naturally and causing stitches, bruising and even more long-term damage to the pelvic floor or perineum that could have been avoided. You're well within your rights to question your doctor (or to get your birth partner to) on his decision. However, you might find that by the time an assisted delivery is mooted, like most women, you're only too grateful for your baby to be helped out in any way possible.

EPISIOTOMY

A word every woman dreads. This is a cut of the perineum and vagina, performed by a midwife or doctor when considered necessary to help your baby make his exit. It's not as horrible as it sounds – at least at the time – as you'll be given an effective form of pain relief in the form of a local anaesthetic injection (unless you've already got an epidural in place).

You'll need to be stitched up again afterwards (as indeed you may be if you tear naturally) and unfortunately this can cause much soreness, itching and discomfort after the birth – not to mention abject fear of having a poo (which can lead to constipation, and an ensuing vicious circle). It should only take a month for stitches to heal completely. They can become infected, though, leading to more misery, and for some women poorly healed stitches can have consequences months down the line. That's why episiotomies are not often carried out these days – most midwives will try their utmost to avoid them. See page 255 for more on your body after birth.

IF YOU NEED AN EMERGENCY CAESAREAN

It's a good idea to know roughly what an emergency caesarean involves, just in case you end up having one. This section will tell you what you need to know, ahead of the possibility.

Sometimes in a labour that has started off normally, an obstetrician may decide that the fastest and safest way to get your baby out is by performing a caesarean section (c-section). For instance, one will probably be mooted if:

- You suddenly develop pre-eclampsia (see page 48)
- Your labour isn't progressing and you're getting exhausted, or your baby has stuck or is becoming distressed.
- Your baby isn't getting the oxygen he needs, or his heartbeat has become irregular.
- A potentially dangerous complication such as placental abruption (see page 67) has occurred.

Mostly, a doctor will have a good reason for wanting to carry out an emergency c-section, and as you won't have much time to get a second opinion, research possible alternatives, or even think it though, you'll have to put your faith in their judgement. However little time there is spare for discussion, though, your doctor must explain his reasoning, and ask for your consent. If you'd planned on or hoped for a normal birth, you might feel disappointed and frightened at being whistled into surgery. You will have to reassure yourself with the knowledge that c-section is a very common surgical procedure – and that, ultimately, giving birth to a healthy baby is what matters, not how you do it.

What happens in a c-section

Once you've given consent for a caesarean to be carried out, you'll be given an anaesthetic. Usually these days, this will be in the form of an epidural. However, in some emergency cases you may need to have a general anaesthetic and if so, your partner won't be able to come to theatre with you. You'll also need a catheter – a tube that empties urine from your bladder – and a drip in your hand, to administer fluids or pain relief when needed.

> **❝** It took longer than we'd anticipated and was much more painful than I'd been led to believe. I'd heard it was meant to be like someone doing washing-up inside you, but it was far worse than that for me, probably because her head was wedged under my ribs and the surgeon had to tug to get her out. **❞**
>
> Jane

Once the anaesthetic's kicked in, an incision is made, usually horizontally across the lower part of the abdomen at the top of the pubic bone or 'bikini line'. It's done this way to avoid weakening the womb muscles, but the added advantage is that the scar won't show from underneath your pubic hair. Very rarely, in certain emergency cases, a 'vertical' cut is made. This action all takes place behind a screen.

A second cut is then made in the uterus so the baby can be lifted out. He'll be handed straight to a paediatrician – who will have been invited along as a matter of routine – to be checked. If he's very small, or poorly, your baby will have to go straight to the special care unit. If not, he can be handed to your birth partner or carefully placed next to you for a cuddle while you're stitched up: this is a major bit of suturing, and takes about half an hour.

If you've had a c-section, it will take you a longer time to recover than a vaginal delivery and if your c-section was an emergency, it's likely to be longer still. There's more on recovery after a c-section on page 261.

> **"** I'd expected it to be a delicate, intricate operation and was surprised by how much thumping and whacking went on on the other side of the blue sheet. But not painful, and all in all a pleasant experience.**"**
> Katie

AFTER THE BIRTH

Your baby's out! Some time soon after you've had your baby – assuming he's well and doesn't need special care – you'll both be taken to a postnatal ward where, more than likely, you'll be left to your own devices for a while. You may want to sleep, but you may still be buzzing and want to spend some time holding, or just staring at your baby.

I can remember feeling quite blown away at this point after my first baby's birth, having been taken up to the post-labour ward in the dead of night. It was almost unreal – a moment I'd so often experienced in my daydreams, now come true. Typically, anxiety struck almost immediately (a feeling that hasn't really let up since) as my daughter was the only baby on the ward who was crying. By daybreak, I'd had about five minutes sleep and I still hadn't quite got my head round the reality – my baby was no longer inside me, but lying next to me in a small plastic hospital cot loudly crying.

Please don't worry if, when you've had your baby, you don't find yourself looking deep into their eyes, convinced you've never loved anything so much in your life. It doesn't always work that way, as *Modern Girl* Nina explains. 'I never bought into that view that once you're holding your baby you forget the pain and fall in love – what a load of bollocks! I'll never forget the pain to my dying day and I couldn't possibly love someone I hadn't got to know. So, although I felt a very strong sense of responsibility and was relieved he was OK, I didn't love him. That came a little later, as we got to know each other and learned to live together.'

Fear is another very common emotion at this moment. 'It's a combination of overwhelming love and terror,' recounts *Modern Girl* Sara. 'I was in a state of physical shock from the delivery, then there was the shock of actually holding my baby for the first time, and it was overwhelming. The baby I'd been trying for for three years was here, no longer a hope or a fantasy but a real, breathing being and I was thrilled by my dream coming true at last, but also terrified by the sudden responsibility. I was shaking like a leaf.'

“ I can't put into words how it feels when your baby is placed on you for the first time. You have to experience it yourself, and even then, you won't be able to describe it to anybody else. It's a mixture of relief, exhaustion, overwhelming love and the realisation that you're going to spend the rest of your life worrying about this little person. It takes even longer to realise that you're actually a mum!**”**
Jenny

10

Birth stories:
six *Modern Girls*
recall their
labour day

These six real birth stories from our *Modern Girls* are not here to scare you, but to show just how diverse people's experiences can be. So do your homework, and be prepared for anything. (Note to very hormonal and overly emotional readers: they might make you cry!)

Judy's birth story

Everything kicked off three weeks early. I suddenly woke up at about 3am and felt weird. I thought about waking up my husband and then I thought, 'He'll ask me what I mean by weird and I can't explain it!' Then I felt something warm trickling down my legs. I woke him up and told him my waters had broken. We called the hospital and they said to go in, but when I got there they said my waters *hadn't* broken – they thought the liquid was just me wetting myself (which apparently can happen when you're heavily pregnant). I wasn't convinced, but thought (as you do) they knew best so I went home again and went to bed.

I carried on 'wetting myself', and then I started getting pains in my back. They started coming about every five minutes, so at about 8am I rang them back and said I *really* thought my waters had gone and as I was having pains in my back could these be contractions? They told me to go in again so we trundled there in the rush-hour traffic. By now I had my TENS machine on as the pains were quite bad.

At the hospital they confirmed my waters *had* gone (er, thanks) and that I was 3cm dilated. I was delighted I'd already got that far but a bit shocked it was happening so early. I was in quite a bit of pain by now but only in my back (yet another thing I hadn't learnt at antenatal classes). They said I could go home but to come back if I needed more pain relief and they booked me in for an induction 24 hours later because my waters had gone. I said I really didn't want to go home as I felt I couldn't cope with much more pain. They examined me and found I was a bit more dilated, so off I went to the labour room.

The pain was getting worse. Gas and air didn't really do the trick so I had a shot of pethidine; which didn't help either. I still only had pains in my back, which was bizarre and not what I was expecting at all. Then the labour just stopped. They decided to induce me and gave me an epidural at the same time as I was knackered (I think it was about 6pm now, but can't be sure) and the contractions would be much stronger. There was talk of a caesarean because they were worried he was getting distressed. But in the end I had him normally – well, if you can count an episiotomy and a ventouse delivery as normal.

He was eventually born at 4.15am and my first thought was, 'Can someone take this baby away so I can get some sleep?' as I was beyond exhausted. The hospital has fantastic sea views, and I remember his dad holding him up to see his first dawn.

Isla's birth story

I had a textbook birth, I suppose. My daughter came on her due date. I felt dull pains throughout the night; emptied my bowels two or three times. I woke up about 7am and thought, 'Hmm, this might be it.' So I sat in a bath for three hours before going to the birthing centre. It was lovely and calm there, the midwives were fantastic, and I had a private room with a shower and toilet. After a six-hour labour, and a bucketful of gas and air, my daughter was born in the pool. I thought the worst bit of the whole thing was having stitches, as I'm queasy.

Jenny's birth story

Unfortunately, our antenatal group was lulled into a false sense of security as the first one of us to give birth went from start to finish in four hours and needed no pain relief or stitches. I started to wonder what the fuss was all about as all I'd heard from other mums was how long and painful it could be. I delivered second out of our group, and let's just say I experienced the other end of the spectrum!

Labour pains started at 5.17am. My other half had spent the week feeding me hot chilli to bring on labour and as I got up to go for a wee, my plug appeared on the bathroom floor. I showed it to my dazed other half and rang the hospital to let them know. They told me to ring back if the pain became more intense and more frequent. It was about 5.40am and there was no way I was getting any more sleep, despite the midwife's advice to. In truth, I was absolutely bricking it.

So, by 6am I was watching a DVD and, for some very bizarre reason, my other half was pruning the hedge in the back garden. He then proceeded to polish the living room and tidy the kitchen. As the morning progressed we started to time the contractions and made regular phone calls to the hospital. By 11am the pain was very intense and I felt I couldn't cope with it any more, so we packed the car and trundled off to the hospital.

When we arrived, I was put into a delivery suite and after a couple of hours, during which I had some gas and air, I was internally checked. This was very invasive and made me cry. I cheered up when my other half had a go at the gas and air while the midwife wasn't in the room, while I took a picture of him. I can only liken gas and air to that feeling you have when you're slightly tipsy. It's great!

On the first inspection I was only 2cm–3cm dilated. Over the next couple of hours I stuck to gas and air and the birthing ball, which was fun, but my dilation was very slow. By 6.30pm, pain was increasing and I got into the birthing pool. It had worked for one of our friends but I found it to be too hot and very uncomfortable.

By now the labour pains were incredibly intense. I was sure I was about to give birth and so was very disheartened to find I was only about 7cm dilated. It was 8.30pm and I'd really had enough. I decided, though I hadn't planned it, to have an epidural.

So I was lugged out of the pool, dried off and put on the bed. Having the epidural was difficult and frightening – the anaesthetist couldn't seem to find the right place on my back and I felt very sick and very scared. It took about 45 minutes for it to kick in. Suddenly, I felt completely normal – the pain had been totally switched off. At 10pm I felt so good I watched *Big Brother*.

At midnight the registrar was called as the baby's heart rate was starting to dip after each contraction and there were signs of meconium. Despite pushing, we weren't getting very far. The registrar gave me an hour to deliver, otherwise it was going to be assisted. At this point, I'd been on the go for 19 hours and was shattered.

I pushed for an hour, but there was no real change, so the registrar returned. She first tried the ventouse cup, which didn't work. So at 1.19am, she performed an episiotomy and used forceps to deliver our daughter, who arrived screaming into the world at 1.22am. She was checked over with the suction to clear any meconium out of her lungs, but she was fine.

For a short time I wasn't interested in our baby and was happy to let her daddy hold her. The midwife later said she'd been worried about this, but it turned out I was having a reaction to the gas and air and epidural, which were making me feel incredibly sick. The midwife gave me an anti-sickness injection and after that I felt fine and wouldn't let my baby go.

My proudest moment came when I was being wheeled into the lift to go to the labour ward, holding my daughter all wrapped up in my arms. This was at 6am, and although I'd been up for over 24 hours and was totally exhausted, the sun was shining on a new day and my baby, who I'd fretted about for nine months, was finally here.

Michelle's birth story

My first baby was due on Valentine's Day. I had a midwife's appointment the day before and was fed up when she said that there was no way the baby was coming soon. But at 6am the next morning my waters broke. I was in no pain at all, but was concerned that the waters seemed an odd colour. Thankfully I had a sample pot in the bathroom and caught some of it. I rang the hospital, as I wasn't having any contractions. They told me to come in as they suspected that the baby had pooed and there was meconium in the water.

I was put on a drip and had a monitor put on me so I couldn't move around. That was pretty horrible. As I was induced the contractions went from nothing to three every 10 minutes. I used gas and air but by mid-afternoon the midwife advised me to have an epidural. That was a joke as it was put in too low, so I couldn't feel my legs but I could feel the contractions.

In the early evening the baby's heartbeat went dangerously low so they put a clip on the top of his head to monitor it, and tested his oxygen levels. That was when there was a decision to have an emergency c-section and I was truly petrified. I so wanted my husband to come with me, but I had to have a general anaesthetic, so he couldn't.

Our son was born at 8.50pm on Valentine's Day. Not the most romantic thing I've ever done, out cold with 20-odd people in the room and my legs up in stirrups! I woke up on a ward at about 11pm to be shown a Polaroid of him, and I finally got to see him in the flesh about three hours later.

Mel's birth story

I had my daughter at home, which friends and family thought I was mad to do. My labour started at 4.30am and my husband filled up the birth pool and got it to the right temperature. We were on our own for most of the time until the midwife came at about noon. Everything was pretty straightforward and I actually fell asleep between contractions when I was in the pool.

In the initial stages I had a TENS machine which was fantastic, but near the end it was annoying me so I went on to gas and air and I had that until she was born an hour or two later.

I felt the urge to push and the head crowned. I felt another big urge so gave it my all and she shot out, hitting the wall of the pool on the other side, much to everyone's surprise. The midwife said to pick the baby up, so I had to fumble about and find her and then picked her up and held her to my chest. After a minute or two the midwife asked me what sex the baby was – I hadn't even looked, I was so busy just staring at it (her). I looked down and said, 'It's a boy!' The midwife, who'd been fantastic, said, 'Actually it's a little girl, that's the umbilical cord!'

I couldn't believe that I'd done it. I was in the pool and holding her for about 10 minutes before we had to get out, just staring into her eyes, thinking she was the most beautiful thing I had seen. The labour was immediately forgotten. It's the most magical feeling in the world.

Unfortunately I had a third-degree tear thanks to her acrobatic exit. It was too big to be stitched at home so we had to transfer to hospital to get it done under an epidural anaesthetic. I have a fear of hospitals and wasn't happy having to stay overnight there. I felt very disappointed that I had done all the hard work at home by myself but had still ended up in hospital having an epidural.

My advice to any mum is to trust your body. You know what's best for you and your baby. If your body is telling you to push, then push. If a position isn't comfortable, try something else. And if you want pain relief, get it. There's no point being a martyr!

Nicola's birth story

I went a week overdue so I went for a sweep and was then advised to go for a long walk, eat some spicy food, and seduce my fella. I went for a four-mile walk and had pasta arrabbiata that night – I didn't bother with the seduction! I woke at 3am with contractions which were 10 minutes apart.

We spent a while on the internet checking to see whether I really was in labour or not and decided I was, so we phoned the hospital. They said to phone back when the contractions were five minutes apart. Andrew gave me a back massage, and we went back to bed. I'd read about a hypnobirthing relaxation technique, which really helped me to relax in between contractions. I got up and had a bath at 6.30am and when I got out I had two more contractions, and phoned my mum. Andrew decided to go back to bed for an hour since we expected it to be a long day, and meanwhile I spent a lot of time sitting on the loo as it was the most comfy place to be. I had a show and diarrhoea during this time.

At 9am Andrew got up and told me to have a paracetamol to ease the pain. I won't repeat what I told him! By now I had backache and my upper legs were tingling. Andrew tried to massage me again, but again I told him where to go. By now I was crawling around the living room on all fours, moaning in pain. I called the labour ward and had a contraction while on the phone to them. They told me to come in straight away because from my voice they could hear I was in the later stages of labour.

We got there at 10am and Andrew parked the car while I staggered to the maternity unit. As soon as I got there my waters broke. The midwife wanted to inspect me but I couldn't get on the bed: it just wasn't comfortable, and she refused to examine me until I was on the bed. Finally I got on – by now my bottom felt as though it was going to explode. The midwife said I was 6cm dilated and they whisked me off to the labour room in a wheelchair. Andrew was still parking the car at this point.

I had a different, nicer midwife then. She told me to get on the bed but again I didn't want to and so she was happy for me to labour standing up. She adjusted the bed so I could lean over it, and gave me gas and air.

Andrew came back and said he'd had to park the car illegally because there were no spaces. The midwife told him I had another three hours to go and advised him to park in an adjacent car park. Then I felt something different downstairs – again, it was as though my bum was going to explode, but worse. I asked the midwife to check how dilated I was again but she said she couldn't as I might get an infection if she checked too often. But I remembered learning in NCT classes that you know your own body best, and if you feel you need to be checked, you should insist. So she checked me again. I was 10cm dilated.

She asked if I wanted to wait for my husband to return before I gave birth and I said I wasn't sure if I could. She told me to get on the bed again but I still didn't want to. I can't explain it, but it just wasn't comfortable sitting or lying down. So she asked if I wanted to have the baby standing up. At that point I could feel a burning sensation and guessed it was the baby's head crowning. Andrew came in after finally parking the car and I asked, 'Where the fuck have you been?'

The midwife told me to push with the pain, but I had no control. We heard a little cry and then whoosh, the baby came out. She caught him, and I saw he was a boy. She injected me with something to make the placenta come out and finally I got on the bed. She gave me Callum straight away and it was lovely. I was delighted and so pleased that Andrew had made it in time, too. It had all been so quick – I'd got to the hospital at 10am and he'd been born just over an hour later. I can only attribute the fact that I delivered standing up to lots of hockey, running and skiing – I've got strong thighs. And I think gravity really does help, too.

11

Hey, baby:
the first few weeks with your newborn

SETTLING IN

It's a really good idea to read this section before you have your baby, for two reasons: one, it's good to be prepared for your headlong plummet into child rearing, and secondly, you won't have time to read anything once he's arrived!

Assuming you had an uncomplicated vaginal delivery, you'll probably be dispatched from the maternity unit within about 12 hours of the birth. Some women just can't wait to get away; others rather enjoy the chance to lie in bed and be tended to for a while.

Once you're all installed at home, with no bustling team of health professionals around, you may well find that anxiety strikes. It can feel weird, too – the fact that all of a sudden, there's another person in the house, relying solely on you and your partner to love it, care for it and make sure it doesn't get damaged. Allow yourself plenty of time to adjust to all this. It's a steep learning curve, and one you need to take at a steady pace.

If you're in any doubt about something, remember you don't have to tackle it alone: put in a call to your midwife or health visitor. If you can't get hold of someone quickly and you feel you need to, you can always call NHS Direct (NHS24 in Scotland). It's a good idea to put all the important telephone numbers somewhere prominent, so you're not scrabbling around in a panic if you need them.

FEEDING YOUR BABY

Getting enough nourishment down your new charge is going to be one of your primary pre-occupations over the coming weeks and months. On page 194 I've covered the pros and cons of breastfeeding and bottlefeeding. I want to reiterate now that how you feed your baby is your choice. There should be no stigma attached to either way.

Breastfeeding: the truth

Lots of women aren't really prepared for what breastfeeding involves, and maybe that's why the early challenges prove too much for so many. Difficulty latching on, severely sore or infected nipples, poor milk supplies, or just a disinterested baby, are all common problems, affecting even the steeliest resolve to feed your baby yourself. Statistics show that three-quarters of UK mums breastfeed initially, but less than a quarter are still giving their baby nothing but breast milk by six weeks, and by six months, the optimum time frame recommended by the Department of Health for breastfeeding, three-quarters have given up on it completely.

❝ My midwife recommended I stay in bed as long as possible and take advantage of a husband who works from home. I lounged in bed for weeks, learning to breastfeed and bond with her – very successfully, too. **❞**
Genevieve

Some other books (and many health professionals) gloss over this bit, but I'm going to be upfront about it: when you're trying to get breastfeeding established, it can really, *really,* hurt. Some people say that if it hurts, you're doing it wrong – but actually, it can hurt if you're doing it right, too (initially, at least), as though someone's attached clamps to your nipples and viciously twisted them. And that's before you develop weals or cracks across the tender skin of your nipples, or worse – an infection – and you then have to put your infected or cracked nipple into the mouth of a hungry baby who will suck on it with no mercy.

The other thing which you're not always warned about breastfeeding is the sheer amount of time you're likely to spend doing it at first. Very young babies don't half do a lot of demanding – feeding so often, and for so long in the early weeks, that it can seem as though you're spending nine–and-a-half out of 10 hours in the day pinned to the sofa.

None of which is intended to be off-putting. The truth is that, once you've got it sussed, breastfeeding becomes a doddle (enjoyable, even). And most early breastfeeding problems *can* be overcome if you're committed, and if you have the right support. So if you're struggling, but determined, ask your midwife or health visitor to help. And if they don't have the time or inclination to help, make contact with a breastfeeding counsellor – there'll be one in your area, or at the very least, on the other end of the phone. There are lots of organisations dedicated to helping with breastfeeding, listed at the back of the book.

❝ Breastfeeding was so hard. Bleeding nipples, a baby who wouldn't latch on and seemed utterly uninterested in feeding made it a complete nightmare. But I was so sure that breast was best I gritted my teeth and got on with it – and within a few weeks we had it sorted. **❞**
Sara

Tips for successful breastfeeding

- Make sure you're comfortable. A footstool and a large pillow under your arm (or better still, a V-shaped breastfeeding cushion) can be a huge help.

- Offer your baby the boob whenever he seems to want it. Although this can be exhausting, it's the best way to keep your supplies up – and it's not for ever. Within a month or two, feeds will become speedier and more widely spaced – honest.

- Make sure your baby gets as big a mouthful of breast as possible. If he's just nibbling away at the end of your nipple he won't be getting the milk out – and you'll be in a lot of pain.

- Take it out and start again if it's wrong. But don't just pull away while he's still sucking for dear life, or you'll be in agony. Pop your little finger in the corner of his mouth to break the suction.

- Let your baby drain the whole breast before offering the other – and go back to that one first at the next feed. (You'll know when it's empty because it will be soft and deflated.) Attach a safety pin or ribbon to your bra strap, and it will help you remember which breast you need to whop out first next time.

- Have lots of breast pads to hand. You won't believe how much milk can leak out.

Hitting the bottle

If you'd decided to bottlefeed or if breastfeeding doesn't take off for some reason and you've decided to go with bottles and formula, don't beat yourself up about it, and ignore any disapproving health professionals or mothers-in-law.

- A natural remedy that really *does* ease sore and engorged boobs is cabbage leaves – although no-one is sure quite why – preferably chilled first in the fridge.

- Don't introduce a bottle or dummy while you're getting breastfeeding established, in case your baby becomes confused.

- If you're shy, you don't have to breastfeed in front of all and sundry. Find a quiet corner or ask for some privacy. A carefully draped muslin will help spare your blushes.

- Keep yourself well fed and watered while you're breastfeeding. Breastfeeding mums need about 400 calories more a day than when they were pregnant – so now you really do have an excuse to eat more. Continue to take 10mcg of vitamin D daily while breastfeeding, for the sake of your baby's bones and teeth.

- Don't smoke if you're breastfeeding, as the nicotine and other dangerous chemicals in tobacco smoke can be passed on to your baby.

- In theory you should stick to the same sort of alcohol limits you did in pregnancy (although, if you can master the art of expressing, you can always freeze supplies of your breast milk, for nights when you fancy a drink or three).

66 I gave her formula from the start. I know breast is best, and all that. But I just had such a problem with the idea of getting my breasts out all the time, and them being sucked on. My little girl has always been happy and healthy, so I really don't think I've harmed her. 99
Kim

As many a mum of a bouncing, bottle-fed baby will tell you, formula's a perfectly good alternative to breast milk, as long as you stick to the rules on hygiene and preparation. And it too has advantages: it doesn't hurt; you can ask someone else to feed your baby for you (a big bonus in the middle of the night); you know exactly how much he's getting; and you won't ever have to get your boobs out in front of your father-in-law. It will also make returning to work a whole lot easier, when the time comes.

A bit of both

Some mums find a happy compromise in mixed feeding – some breast-feeds, some formula. Introducing a bottle tends to be easier the earlier you do it – hardly surprisingly, perhaps, as once a baby's accustomed to drinking sweet, warm breastmilk from a nice, soft boob, a rubber-teat and fake-tasting formula probably doesn't have the same appeal – so you might have to be persistent when it comes to introducing one. Once you've done so, though, you should find your baby will happily take from both – you can decide for yourself which feeds you want to be bottle and which breast, but you'll need to stick to the same method at the same times of the day, because of the supply and demand nature of the way the boobs work. One word of warning about mixed feeding, though: your boobs will quickly adjust to any new routine and a decreased demand. So if you start it, you'll fairly soon get to a point where you can't go back.

66 I really wanted to breastfeed and persisted for six weeks with a baby who lost weight and was permanently grumpy. Finally I switched to formula and overnight he went from

being the grumpiest baby in the world to a complete angel. This was when the penny dropped that he was probably cross because I'd been starving him. Doh!**"**
Nina

YOUR POST-BIRTH BODY

This is probably high on your list of worries – how on earth does your body return to normal after such an ordeal? Usually it will depend on what kind of birth you had. Some women get off lightly and find they recover within weeks. For others, it may take months. To one degree or another, though, you're going to feel knackered and sore. And there are a whole host of other things your poor old body might have to cope with, too.

" I thought you were meant to feel better after nine months of pregnancy. I was looking forward to sleeping on my front, getting my tummy back and generally feeling myself again. Unfortunately I had infected stitches, and mastitis, so for six weeks I was in agony. As for sleeping on your front – when your milk comes in it's the last thing you want to do.**"**
Jo

Bleeding

Known as lochia, the postnatal discharge of blood, mucus and tissue as the womb sheds its lining is experienced by every new mother. It varies from woman to woman, but you might find the amount somewhat alarming. 'I was really shocked by the aftermath,' recalls *Modern Girl* Rebecca. 'Oh man, the amount of bleeding. It just seemed like there was blood everywhere for weeks.'

Lochia is usually very heavy and bright red in colour for a few days but becomes lighter, changing to brown or pink, and will normally stop altogether within six weeks. If it returns to a bright red colour at any point, mention it to your midwife, as it could be a sign of infection, or that you're overdoing things. You'll need plenty of maternity pads to cope with the flow – tampons aren't a good idea because they could introduce infection into the vagina and normal sanitary towels probably won't be up to the job. You should definitely tell your midwife if the bleeding doesn't slow after a few weeks, if it suddenly becomes extremely heavy or repeatedly clotted (some clots are normal), or if it starts to smell, as this could signal a problem.

Afterpains

Thought you'd felt your last contraction for a while during the birth? Erm, no, sorry – there's a few more to come. Your womb has to contract back to its normal size in the days after birth and this can be painful, particularly while breastfeeding, as it releases oxytocin, the hormone that triggers contractions. A painkiller such as paracetamol can help, as can a heat pack, or hot water bottle.

Vagina and perineum

If you tore or had an episiotomy, you're going to be very sore indeed down below, and even if you didn't, it's likely to feel bruised and tender for a while – a fact you'll be painfully reminded of every time you sit down, or attempt to walk anywhere, probably in the manner of John Wayne. 'My nether regions felt like a bomb had gone off down there. It took about three months before it felt anything like normal,' admits *Modern Girl* Nina.

If you had stitches, these may give you quite a bit of grief, with itchiness as well as pain compounding the misery. You can buy a range of products to help ease this discomfort, such as gel-filled packs which you chill and then pop in your pants, and anaesthetic sprays. Plain old painkillers and warm baths will usually offer relief, and some women reckon a drop or two of an appropriate essential oil such as lavender or teatree can help, too. Arnica is widely believed to help relieve bruising and inflammation and boost the healing process, and some women swear by it. You can buy it in health food shops and most chemists, but make sure you read the label carefully before taking. And if sitting is a sore point, you could look into hiring a specially designed, inflatable 'valley cushion'. The NCT and some private companies offer these for hire.

Stitches can become infected, so your midwife will check them several times during her home visits to make sure they're healing without any problems. Try to keep the area clean – use a handheld shower to rinse it a couple of times a day, especially after using the loo. Try using tissues rather than a towel, or even use a hairdryer (gives a whole new meaning to the term 'wash and blow dry …') Change your pad regularly, making sure you wash your hands before and after. Stitches will usually dissolve on their own after a week or two, but sometimes they may need to be taken out.

Soreness down below makes going to the loo after birth a major trial. Having a wee can sting like buggery – it helps to tinkle just before you get out of the bath, or pour warm water over your bits in mid-flow. Drink plenty of fluids, as this will reduce the concentration of your urine and make it sting less.

Doing your pelvic floor exercises will help healing, as it increases blood flow to the area, so do get cracking on these as soon as you can bear. Turn back to page 122 to remind yourself how.

It's a grim thought, but if you're unlucky enough to experience a very bad tear (known as a third- or fourth-degree tear), you could end up suffering from bladder and bowel problems. Pelvic floor exercises will be particularly important, and you can be referred to an obstetric physiotherapist for specialist help.

Assuming everything's OK, you'll get the go-ahead from your doctor to have sex again six weeks after birth (although it's all right to try before that, if you're in good shape below, your lochia flow has ceased – and you can find the energy). In reality, many women don't feel up to it, for psychological as well as physical reasons, for several months or more.

You might also worry about the way your vagina looks and feels after childbirth, perhaps fearing you've been left with something of a 'wizard's sleeve' down there. It's true that elasticity can be reduced, and that raised scar tissue may have changed its appearance, which can make things feel and look a little different down there. But most couples find these to be minor details. If you're really worried that things aren't right, have a chat to your GP.

Bowels and bum

Trying to do a poo in the days after birth can become a trauma of rather large proportions, not helped by the fact that the bowels can become sluggish after birth, anyway, because the muscles and nerves down there have come in for such a bashing. 'By *far* the worst post-birth issue I had was having a poo,' recounts *Modern Girl* Lara. 'I was ridiculously scared about it – mainly I think because I was worried about bursting my stitches – and of course the longer I left it, the more scared I got.'

In fact, it's highly unlikely you'll rip open your stitches, but it might feel as if you're going to. Holding a maternity pad or a clean wedge of tissues over the stitches should give you the psychological reassurance you need to go for it. Constipation will make things worse (and this can lead to a bit of a vicious circle), so keep up your fibre intake and drink plenty of water. If necessary, ask your midwife to recommend a gentle laxative treatment. And bear in mind that, although many women dread the first bowel movement, in reality it probably won't be as bad as you fear.

Piles are common after birth, caused by the pressure of the delivery on your anus, and can make for yet more painful, itchy misery. You can buy over-the-counter treatments which offer some relief, and if they're really bad your midwife will be able to get a suppository prescribed for you. But they should go away on their own after a while.

Boobs

A couple of days after birth, your milk 'comes in', and you will wake up to discover that you have two unbearably tender breasts suddenly the size and texture of granite boulders. It's caused by a big hormonal surge, and won't last longer than a couple of days.

If you're breastfeeding, the best way to relieve the pain and pressure this causes is to feed your baby – although you may find you have to gently express a little at first (try massaging them while you're in the bath) so they're not too full for him to get his mouth round. And yes, it's an irony: the biggest boobs you've ever had and the only person reaping the benefits is your baby. That's life.

Do let your midwife know if any red patches appear on your breast, and/or you're suffering from flu-like symptoms: this could be a sign of mastitis, a condition that causes the breast tissue to inflame painfully and may need treatment.

If you're not breastfeeding, there'll be a painful few days while the milk subsides (and it should have dried up completely within a few weeks). You'll need a snug-fitting bra, and possibly some paracetamol, to ease your way through this period.

> **"** I'd gone from a 32DD to a 34F during pregnancy. Once the milk came in four days after the birth I woke up with 34HH Zeppelins attached to my chest. They remained that way for about four months. I am 5ft tall. How I stood up, I don't know. **"**
> Sheridan

Belly

Your tummy will still be big for a while, only it won't be firm and round any more, it'll be as wobbly as blancmange. Don't whatever you do worry about this during the first few months – there'll be time enough in the future to get back into your old jeans – and it's certainly not a good idea to start working out before the first six weeks. However, if you want to make a tentative start on getting some strength back in your abdomen, you can, by gently pulling in your tummy and holding it for a few seconds before releasing, whenever you get the chance.

As for stretch marks, if you have them, they'll fade eventually – although they won't go altogether. There are lots of lotions and potions on the market at varying prices that claim to help, but since none are proven to have dramatic effects, you may as well stick to inexpensive cocoa butter or vitamin E-based brands if you're keen to give one a go. Meanwhile, lots of women swear by fake tan as a means of covering up the worst of their 'baby battlescars'.

If your stretch marks are really bad and are getting you down, however, it's worth chatting to your GP about it as there are a couple of stronger treatment creams available and he may be willing to prescribe one for you. If you're truly desperate – and have the financial clout – you could look at either laser treatment or cosmetic surgery, but talk to your doctor first.

Serious post-birth symptoms

There are some post-pregnancy symptoms that could signal a serious complication, so don't hesitate to give your midwife or GP a shout if your bleeding becomes very severe; if you feel faint, dizzy or feverish; there's any swelling or tenderness or pain in your legs; you can't shake a severe headache, particularly if it comes with vomiting or blurred vision; you have a persistent pain in the tummy or down below, or you're having a lot of pain when weeing.

Weak or leaky bladders

Don't be surprised if you're finding it hard to keep urine in – weak and leaky bladders are another common and delightful consequence of giving birth. Doing your pelvic floors exercises will help (everyone should do them after birth, anyway, to avoid problems in the future). And you're not excused just because you had a c-section – pregnancy in itself puts a strain on your pelvic floor, so you could still be at risk. If the problem's really bad, or persists beyond a few weeks, tell your doctor. They may refer you to a specialist for treatment. I have to say, my bladder has never been the same since I had babies. I suppose I must just be grateful I didn't get the stretch marks.

> **❝** I was expecting to be in huge amounts of discomfort, pain and general yuckiness. While I did spend the first couple of days feeling pretty uncomfortable, I was pleasantly surprised at how quickly everything healed and how little actual pain there was. **❞**
>
> Lara

RECOVERY AFTER A CAESAREAN SECTION

A caesarean section is major abdominal surgery, and so it will usually take longer to recover from than a vaginal birth. How long that will be varies. You should have got over the worst after six weeks, but some women say they still don't feel right for up to a year afterwards. Recovery from an emergency c-section is likely to take longer then if you had an elective.

- You'll have to stay in hospital for three to four days, on average, and you'll need some heavy-duty painkilling medication. You'll be given a good supply of pain relief medication to take home with you, too.

- You'll probably find even simple activities like sitting up and walking hard work, and will need lots of help and support in doing so (if you're on your own, you may need a good friend or relative to come and stay with you for a while).

- There's no reason why you can't cuddle and breastfeed your baby – although you may need a little help in working out how to do so comfortably.

- Whilst you're still in hospital, you'll see a physiotherapist. She'll help you to get walking again, and will show you some exercises that will keep the circulation going in your legs and so prevent the formation of a blood clot (see page 44) and you'll probably be asked to wear a rather fetching pair of compression stockings, for the same reason.

- As it will hurt to cough or laugh, she'll show you to do so without it causing trouble for your incision site.

- It's common to suffer from painful trapped wind after a caesarean, as your digestive system may have been affected by the surgery. Peppermint tea is widely recommended as a means of relief.

- Don't panic if your incision site looks very obvious or vivid at this point – it will shrink and fade to a fine, pale line with time. You may suffer from some itchiness around the area and it's a good idea to keep it clean and dry. The stitches will either dissolve or need removing at a later stage.

- Dress in very loose comfortable clothing for a while. In particular, you're going to need some very roomy pants.

- You'll be warned not to drive for at least a couple of weeks after a having a c-section (although your insurance company may insist on six – check the small print) and to avoid lifting anything heavy for several months.

- Sometimes, women who've had an unplanned, emergency c-section find it hard to deal with emotionally. They might be disappointed because they didn't get the natural birth they planned, or even that they've 'failed' to have a 'proper' birth. One way to deal with this is to go over what happened during the birth. (See below).

> **❝** I found the c-section debilitating. I couldn't get out of bed to get to the toilet, or stand up next to my babies to change their nappies, and I have never felt so much pain. I hated the experience, but in hindsight I know it was the best thing for their health, and mine. A year on I still have twinges from my scar. I tell you, it's the best contraception a girl can have because I am not doing that again. **❞**

Amanda

YOUR POSTNATAL CARE

In most areas you'll remain under the care of a community midwife for around 10 days, and she should arrange to drop in on you several times during this period to make sure both you and your baby are doing OK, after which your health visitor – a qualified nurse or midwife who works in the community with families – will take over. Exactly how many visits you get will depend on policy, how pressed they are, and how much you need them.

Your baby should get a full medical once-over within three days of his birth – this could either be when you're still in hospital or once you get home, usually by a visiting GP. His height and weight measurements will be taken, and checks made on his eyes, hearts, hips, and (boys only, naturally) testes. A week or so after the birth, your midwife will want to take a heel prick test on your newborn. It's a routine screening process which involves taking a small sample of blood from your baby's heel, which is then sent away to check for a number of rare but serious conditions. Your baby will also be offered vitamin K, either in the form of a single injection or two or three separate oral doses, which protects against another very rare but dangerous condition, vitamin K deficiency bleeding (VKDB). And these days, all babies get a routine hearing test soon after birth, too – it's a very quick, simple test that involves a small earpiece being put in your baby's ear for a few moments.

Your midwife will want to make sure you're doing OK too. When she comes, she'll examine your belly to make sure your womb is returning to normal, and check your stitches to see if they're healing and there's no sign of infection. She'll look at your legs for signs of a blood clot (see page 44); check your temperature and blood pressure; and make sure your blood loss is normal. She'll also want to know that your bowel and

The alien has landed

Wondering if you had in fact given birth to an alien – or which one of you he inherited that strange shaped head from? Fear not. Newborn babies are weird little beings, with many mysterious features. Here are some random facts about them that may surprise you:

- Their first poos (meconium) are dark and sticky. The dark sticky stuff will soon give way to something yellow or green and runny (in breastfed babies) but paler and firmer (and generally smellier) if formula-fed.

- Their skin is very often flaky, blotchy, rashy or spotty. (Check with your health visitor if you're worried, but in most cases it will be harmless and normal.)

- They may be very hairy. This is the remains of lanugo, the covering that protected them in the womb, and will drop out soon.

- They may also still have vernix on them, and so be a bit greasy. Don't bother trying to wash it off, it'll help protect against dry skin.

- Their heads may be a weird shape, squished by the journey down the birth canal (and especially if vacuum extraction or forceps were used to ease him out). The soft spot on the top, where the skull bones have yet to fuse, is called the fontanelle. It's likely to be a year bladder movements are OK. She may ask you about contraception and although your immediate reaction may be to snort with laughter, it's worth bearing in mind, since it's technically possible to conceive just three weeks after giving birth – even if you *are* breastfeeding.

Both you and your baby will also be offered a more comprehensive check-up, usually with a GP or practice nurse, six to eight weeks after the birth.

or more before it closes up. In the meantime, you don't have to be neurotic about damaging it – there's a tough layer of membrane underneath the skin which you'd really have to go some to penetrate.

- Their eyes may squint. This is because the muscles around them have yet to develop.

- The remains of the umbilical cord stays attached to their bellies for a few weeks after birth, after which it shrivels and drops off, leaving you with a delightful souvenir of their early weeks. In the meantime, keep a careful eye and let your midwife or health visitor know if it looks sore, as it can sometimes become infected.

- Their genitals and nipples may be swollen, due to hormones passed on by you. If you have a little girl, she may have a little blood in her nappy for the same reason.

- They are very likely to chuck up a large amount of milk when you feed them. This is known as possetting. It's normal, but check with your health visitor if it seems truly copious, is projectile or a strange colour, or they seem to be in pain.

- They may sleep for hours and hours on end during the day in the first few weeks. Make the most of the time to catch up on some rest yourself!

BABYCARE ESSENTIALS

“ I must admit to being baffled by newborn care. I had never held a baby before and it really showed. We made so many mistakes it was farcical. But she's still alive and she's now a happy, healthy child who's unscathed by the ordeals her inept parents put her through. **”**
Sara

This is, as you've hopefully gathered, a pregnancy book. But here's a very basic outline of baby care essentials so you can read, prepare and digest this info before the baby comes.

Washing your baby

There's no reason why you can't put your baby in the big bath from the start, but as this can sometimes freak them out a little at first, you might be better off just to 'top and tail' them in the early weeks. You don't even need a baby bath for this: a clean washing-up bowl of cooled, boiled water will do just fine. Undress him, wrap in a towel to keep warm, and then gently wipe his eyes, face, neck and around the ears (not inside), around the cord stump, hands and nappy area. Watch out in particular for dribbles of milk gathering in folds under the neck and armpits – some babies have been known to produce cheese under here! Dry him, creases too, by gently patting with a towel.

Changing your baby

Put a new nappy on your baby straight away after he's done a poo, or whenever it's getting a bit soggy, to help prevent nappy rash. Clean and dry his bottom thoroughly (cotton wool and water's usually recommended, but alcohol-free baby wipes won't cause any harm), and apply a little barrier cream. It's important to keep a close eye on their bottom business: wet nappies are a good sign he's feeding well: generally speaking, he should be producing six to eight wees over 24 hours. As for poo, the habits of breastfed babies can be wildly erratic, and it's nothing to worry about if they go for several days without one; while formula-fed babies are more prone to constipation, so you should mention it to a health visitor or midwife if yours hasn't done a poo for more than a day.

Holding your baby

It's normal to feel scared about this at first, since new babies are just so small, floppy and delicate. You'll soon work out how he most likes to be held, but meanwhile, the most important thing to remember is to support their heads, as they have no strength in their neck muscles for the first few months.

66 It's not instinctive, caring for your first baby. I used to think his head would fall off at the slightest provocation. He refused to be held cradle style, despite people telling me how to do it 'properly'. He loved being upright over shoulders. You should go with what you discover for yourself, not what people tell you. **99**
Sheridan

Why won't he stop crying?

Some parents are flabbergasted by how much their new baby cries – between one and three hours a day of wailing is quite normal – and, very often, it's for no discernible reason. I myself have had two criers – hence the haunted look in my eyes that lingers there still.

Though mystifying and distressing, it's not unusual to have a baby who cries excessively – up to a fifth of babies are believed to suffer from the tendency (although frankly, it's the parents who come off worst). Excessive crying is usually called colic. No-one's really sure why exactly it happens, although there are plenty of theories – the most popular is that it's due to pain caused by an immature digestive system, although some say it's the baby freaking out as the reality of life outside the womb hits home, and others suggest it's a reaction to uptight parenting (which in my case, explains a lot).

If your baby's crying relentlessly, it's important first to rule out any possible triggers by checking he's not hungry, tired, in need of a feed, or poorly. If it's none of those things, then all you can do is work your way through a list of potential solutions, which will usually include holding, cuddling, jiggling, rocking, swinging, or singing. Sometimes, a walk in the pushchair or sling can work wonders. Other times, a drive in the car is the only thing that can help. And many parents swear by a vibrating chair. There are various commercial preparations, such as Infacol, which are said to help with colic – these won't definitely help, but you may feel it's worth a shot. Some theorise that baby massage or cranial osteopathy – an alternative therapy that involves the application of light pressure, in an attempt to reduce tension within the body – are the answer.

Do check with your health visitor or GP if you have a problem with a relentlessly crying baby, as once in a while, there'll be a medical reason for their distress. However, in most cases, you'll probably be told to grin and bear it. Please believe me when I say it's a short-term problem: it *will* stop, and your sanity *will* return. The good news about colic is that it almost always eases up by the time your baby is about three months old, which is not so long in retrospect (although it's true that it may as well be three years if you're in the thick of it).

❝ I remember once she was crying and crying when I was holding her and for a very brief second I felt like throwing her down and away from me. I laid her gently down in her cot and went outside for some air, and I was fine after that – thank God. But I'll never forget that feeling and it scared me. **❞**

Isla

If in doubt, walk out

It's normal to have feelings of anger and desperation sometimes, if you have a baby who cries a lot. And I know only too well – I've been there. Twice. When you get to a point where you've reached the end of your tether, try to enlist help from someone else until you can feel calm again – or, if there's no-one around, put your baby in his cot and leave the room for a few moments and take some deep breaths. Make yourself a cup of tea, or pour a glass of wine. Phone a friend if need be. He'll come to no harm left crying for a short period. And when you need a break; you need a break.

Now you know what they mean by sleepless nights ...

When they're not feeding, new babies usually sleep (let's face it there's not much else to do, really, at that age). Unfortunately, this pattern of sleeping/feeding just carries on over 24 hours, so that day isn't really any different from night. You can fully expect to be woken four or more times by a new baby wanting sustenance. There's not a lot to be done about it, but pander to the wee insomniac's needs. Things do settle down and night wakings will (usually) become less frequent over the coming months. And later still, when your baby is five or six months old, there are techniques that will help him sleep through the whole night. Until then, you'll just have to accept you're going to be a walking zombie for a while.

> 66 My God, I've never ever felt so tired in my life. Some days, I couldn't string a sentence together. You do forget about this tiredness though – especially when your baby is nine months old and mostly sleeping 11 hours a night (yes, it does happen!) 99
> Jenny

269

Safe sleeping

Cot death is rare, thankfully. But 300 babies a year still die suddenly and unexpectedly in their sleep. No-one knows for certain why, but there are a great many factors that increase the risk, and lots of measures you can take to reduce it. In a nutshell, though, the golden rules are:

- Put your baby to sleep on his back.

- Make up his bedding at the foot of the cot (so he can't wriggle down under his covers).

- Make sure he's not overdressed (a single vest and sleepsuit's fine), and the room isn't too hot (16-20°C is ideal – you can get a room thermometer for a few quid from FSID, but they're often given free with baby magazines or when you buy other equipment).

- Don't put too much bedding on – one blanket's usually enough.

- Don't fall asleep with your baby on a sofa or chair and think carefully before having your baby in bed with you. (Most experts advise against bed-sharing in any circumstances, but if you really want to have your baby in bed with you, make sure you follow the guidelines given by UNICEF which aim to minimise the risks: don't bed-share if one or both of you smoke; if either of you has been drinking or taking any other mind-altering substance; if your baby is very small or was premature; or if you are 'unusually' tired. If in doubt, talk to your midwife or health visitor.)

- Don't smoke near your baby – or anywhere in the house. (Carbon monoxide is exhaled on the breath for several hours following each cigarette and there's a very strong link between smoking and cot death. If you haven't given up by now, you really should.)

- Keep your baby's crib or cot in your room with you, for the first six months.

HOW YOU'LL FEEL

There's a general view that once you've had a baby, life is sweet. It certainly can be. But it's normal to feel a real mixed bag of emotions initially, with lows as common as the highs. An attack of the 'baby blues' affects the vast majority of women during the early days after birth and while these are often blamed on a surge of hormones, they're just as likely to be a simple reaction to an exhausting birth experience or overwhelming change. Baby blues pass quickly and are best tackled with rest, cuddles, and a good cry. But keep an eye on them: for up to one in five women they may give way to postnatal depression, a more serious condition which typically kicks in a month or two down the line, and can take a severe emotional toll.

Also far beyond the mild ups and downs of baby blues is birth trauma, which can occasionally affect women who are left seriously shaken by birth itself and is considered by experts to be a form of post-traumatic stress disorder. If this is something that affects you, do confide in a sympathetic health professional, as it's really important that you get some help with it. Talking through your birth experience is reckoned to be a positive thing to do – your hospital may offer a service that allows you to go in and get any 'unresolved feelings' (often known as 'debriefing' or 'birth reflections') off your chest; or, you may be able to get some counselling.

Bonding with your baby

It's not always love at first sight. Plenty of new mums look down at the baby they've just produced and feel pretty blank. As *Modern Girl* Rebecca remembers: 'I didn't bond instantly with my daughter. I was too shocked, tired and clueless to, I guess. It took me weeks and weeks – perhaps even months.' It's a sentiment echoed by Lara. 'I was expecting the instant rush of love that you read about, but I can honestly say that didn't happen – possibly a side effect of a four-day labour and an epidural!' she says. 'But about 24 hours later I looked over at her, fast asleep in her hospital crib, and cried tears of happiness. And that was when I got the rush of love.'

Give yourself time – you'll almost certainly be flooded with feelings of love for your baby at some point, soon. If not, then don't be afraid to talk to your midwife about it. It could be that you're suffering from postnatal depression and for that, you'll need some kind of help.

> 66 Despite having a miserable time of it after the birth, bonding with my little girl was the easy bit. From the moment she was born I fell in love with her. 99
>
> Jo

Taking it easy

The best piece of advice I can give you is to take it easy straight after you've had your baby. You've got a lot on your plate, what with the physical recovery from birth, and the emotional adjustment to parenthood to make. Lean on your partner and/or anyone else who's around and is willing to give you support at this time. Let the housework go (although a little attention to basic hygiene is probably sensible) and eat ready meals and snacks if you need to.

Visitors will obviously be keen to come and you may well be happy to see them. But don't offer to cook for them (ask them to bring *you* food) and don't be afraid to politely impose a time limit on their stay. Obviously if it's a good friend or a close relative who you enjoy having around and who's prepared to make themselves useful, then that's fine. On the other hand, if a mother-in-law from hell is making your life miserable by staring at you every time you try to breastfeed, or offering unsolicited advice that you could, frankly, do without, you should probably ask them to leave – or give them an 'important' job to do in a different room.

Above all, spend this time getting to know your baby and make the most of this undeniably special period in your baby's life. Before you know it, he's going to be a hulking great toddler, ripping your house apart at the seams and challenging your parenting skills with a whole new set of unfathomable behaviours. Enjoy him while he can't answer back. And good luck.

Useful contacts

General information and support

Bounty parenting club: www.bounty.com

For new and expectant parents: www.babycentre.co.uk

Information on pregnancy and motherhood: www.emmasdiary.co.uk; www.bounty.com; www.babycente.com

Websites for mum: www.netmums.com; www.mumsnet.com

National Childbirth Trust (NCT): www.nctpregnancyandbabycare.com

Pregnancy and birth helpline: 0300 3300 772

Royal College of Obstetricians and Gynaecologists: www.rcog.org.uk

Midwives Online: www.midwivesonline.com

NHS Choices: www.nhs.uk

NHS Direct (for England and Wales): 0845 4647

NHS24 (for Scotland): 08454 242424

Support for lone parents

Campaigning charity: www.gingerbread.org.uk; 0800 018 5026

Survival guide: www.singlemumsurvivalguide.co.uk

Screening and abnormalities

NHS foetal anomaly screening programme: www.fetalanomaly. screening.nhs.uk

Information and support for Down's syndrome parents: www.downs-syndrome.org.uk; 0845 230 0372

Antenatal testing: www.arc-uk.org; 020 7631 0285

Group B Strep support: www.gbss.org.uk; 01444 416176

Medical conditions

Thrombosis: www.thrombosis-charity.org.uk; 020 7633 9937

Pre-eclampsia: www.apec.org.uk; 020 8427 4217

Obstetric Cholestasis: www.ocsupport.org.uk

Pelvic girdle pain: www.pelvicpartnership.org.uk; *01235 820921*

Association of Chartered Physiotherapists in Women's Health: www. acpwh.org.uk

Losing a baby

Ectopic pregnancy: www.ectopic.org.uk; 020 7733 2653

Miscarriage: www.miscarriageassociation.org.uk; 01924 200799

Alcohol and smoking

Information and advice on alcohol consumption: www.drinkaware.co.uk

Online help to quit smoking: www.smokefree.gov

Pregnancy Smoking Helpline: 0800 169 9 169

Food safety

Health in pregnancy, including diet and nutrition: www.tommys.org; Pregnancy Information Service: 0870 777 3060

Eating for Pregnancy: www.eatingforpregnancy.co.uk; 0845 130 3646

Food Standards Authority: www.eatwell.gov.uk

British Dietetic Association: www.bda.uk.com

Exercise

Guild of pregnancy and postnatal exercise instructors: www.postnatalexercise.co.uk

Employment

Health and Safety Executive: www.hse.gov.uk/mothers; 0845 345 0055

Directgov, official government website: www.direct.gov.uk

Acas, employment relations service: www.acas.org.uk; 08457 47 47 47

Department for Work and Pensions: www.dwp.gov.uk

Working Families, helps establish home and work balance: www.workingfamilies.org.uk; 0800 013 0313

Russell Jones and Walker, solicitors: www.rjw.co.uk; 0800 916 9015

Childcare

National Childminders Association: www.ncma.org.uk; 0800 169 4486

National Day Nurseries Association: www.ndna.org.uk; 01484 40 70 70

Relationships

Relate: www.relate.org.uk; 0300 100 1234

The Parent Connection: www.theparentconnection.org.uk

Birth

Where to have your baby: www.birthchoiceuk.com

Home birth: www.homebirth.org.uk

Association for Improvements in the Maternity Services: www.aims.org.uk

Independent Midwives: www.independentmidwives.org.uk; 0845 4600 105

Reflexology: www.aor.org.uk; 01823 351010

Aromatherapy: www.aromatherapycouncil.co.uk

Acupuncture: www.acupuncture.org.uk; 020 8735 0400

Hypnotherapy: www.hypnobirthing.co.uk; www.natalhypnotherapy.co.uk

Doulas: www.doula.org.uk; 0871 4333103

Information and support on all aspects of caesareans: www.caesarean.org.uk

Caesarean procedure and mother's rights information: www.csections.org

Induction information: www.labourinduction.co.uk

Multiple births

Twins and Multiple Birth Association: www.tamba.org.uk; 0800 138 0509

Premature and poorly babies

Special care baby charity: www.bliss.org.uk; 0500 618 140

Breastfeeding

NCT breastfeeding helpline: 0300 330 0771

La Leche League Helpline: 0845 120 2918

National Breastfeeding Helpline: 0300 100 0212

Safety

Foundation for the Study of Infant Death Syndrome: www.fsid.org.uk

Child Accident Prevention Trust: www.capt.org.uk

INDEX